# Baby's Best Chance

## a perinatal manual for parents

**Province of British Columbia**
Ministry of Health
COMMUNITY HEALTH

## PLEASE NOTE

The editors have taken the liberty of using "he" and "him" when referring to the baby and physician. It was decided not to use "she/he, him/her" for the sake of brevity and maintaining continuity of thought.

This book is free to expectant parents in B.C.
Extra copies may be obtained for $3.00 from
Health Promotion and Information
British Columbia Ministry of Health
1515 Blanshard Street
Victoria, B.C.
V8W 3C8

# PREFACE

The need for Baby's Best Chance was recognized by the Perinatal Programme of the British Columbia Medical Association, the metropolitan health services for the Vancouver and Victoria areas and the provincial health units within the Ministry of Health. As a result, copies of the Boundary and Simon Fraser Health Units' Perinatal Manuals and the booklet, *Healthy Mothers Make Healthy Babies* (prepared by the Nova Scotia Department of Health), were distributed to all health units to determine the content appropriate for a provincial manual.

From these suggestions, a draft was prepared by the committee members* and circulated to all public health units who obtained comments from interested staff, hospital personnel, physicians, parents and community representatives throughout the province. The final copy was prepared and edited by the Division of Public Health Nursing in cooperation with Dr. Patricia Baird of the Health Surveillance Registry, Miss Donna Gunther of the Dental Division, Dr. H.K. Kennedy of the Division of Venereal Disease Control and Miss Jane Noble of the Nutrition Division, all of the British Columbia Ministry of Health.

Special recognition is given to Dr. Sydney Segal, Professor of Pediatrics and Head, Division of Maternal, Fetal and Neonatal Medicine of the University of British Columbia, for his cooperation and assistance in the production of the final version and for having suggested the title for this book.

It is seldom that a book is written with input from so many individuals. In checking sources and different opinions, the editors recognized that many differing views exist among the most authoritative persons. Consequently, many of the issues in this book are controversial and highlight the need for discussion and research.

In view of the number of contributors to the original drafts and to the many who made thoughtful and indepth reviews, it is not possible to recognize each contributor individually, but without this cooperation Baby's Best Chance could not have been made possible.

If inadvertently, any reference has been omitted from the bibliography the editors would appreciate being informed.

The editors wish to thank Mr. M. Chazottes, Executive Director, Health Promotion and Information and his staff for their cooperation and the summer students who have assisted in preparing this book. Special thanks must go also to the secretaries for their help and Miss L. Crane, Director of Public Health Nursing, for her patience and support in this undertaking.

Margaret Wilson B.S.N., M.N., M.P.H.
Beulah I. Moricky B.N., M. Sc.N.
Division of Public Health Nursing

March/79

# TABLE OF CONTENTS

Page

# CHAPTER 1

# THE EXPECTANT MOTHER'S TEAM

The expectant mother is not alone in the great adventure of child-bearing. There are a number of team members who are available to help her throughout pregnancy, birth and the postnatal period. The team includes the father or father substitute (referred to throughout the book as the father), physician, dentist, hospital and health unit staff members. Some of the team members and their roles are depicted below.

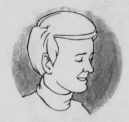

**FATHER**
Emotional Support
Communication Expert
Assistant — Labor
And Delivery
Lover

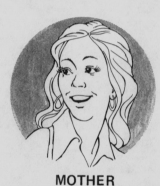

**MOTHER**

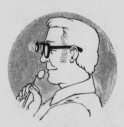

**PHYSICIAN**
Diagnosis
Counselling
Monitoring
Delivery
Supervision

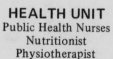 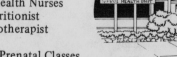

**HEALTH UNIT**
Public Health Nurses
Nutritionist
Physiotherapist

- Prenatal Classes
- Hospital Liaison
- Postnatal Classes
- Home Visiting
- Child Health Conferences

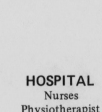 

**HOSPITAL**
Nurses
Physiotherapist
Dietitian

- Labor and Delivery
- Postpartum Care
- Nursery Care

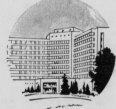

**DENTIST**
Check-up
Teaching
Treatment

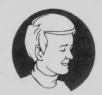

## The Father's Role:

For many years, the baby's father was the forgotten factor during the pregnancy and his place at the time of labor and delivery was thought to be "the further away the better". Fortunately, today, these attitudes have changed and he is recognized as an asset in the pregnancy, during the birth process and throughout the adjustment phase at home. Being the most significant member of the support team, the father provides love, encouragement, companionship and guidance for his partner.

Pregnancy can be a time of increased stress and worry for the father. He may even develop some symptoms of pregnancy. One of his concerns may be the possible loss of income if mother is working and will have to stop. There are baby supplies to purchase, living quarters may need alterations or the family may have to move.

Emotionally, the father must face the fact that his wife's attention will be divided, and that household duties may have to be allocated differently. It is important to recognize these changes so that both parents can work out solutions during the course of the pregnancy.

Staff in many hospitals welcome the father as a reassuring, familiar person to be with the mother throughout labor and delivery. The emotional support he provides can reduce the mother's need for medication in labor and, as indicated in the labor guide section, page 57, the father can be of great help in assisting his partner through the first and second stages of labor. Moreover, by helping in this way, he shares in the child's birth, making the experience meaningful for the whole family.

When a baby is to be born by caesarian section in the operating room, it is wise to find out the physician's and hospital's policies about father's attendance.

Now the father is no longer "the forgotten man" and hopefully over the next few years, his participation will increase and the advantages of his involvement will be more clearly appreciated.

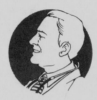

## The Physician:

Most pregnancies are healthy. Problems can be anticipated or prevented by the physician and complications can be reduced to a minimum. But to do this, the doctor needs to know a great deal about the mother and family so that he can make an accurate assessment. He will ask about the mother's personal and family history, and make a careful physical examination, including blood and urine tests. He may also arrange for other diagnostic procedures.

Both future parents should visit the doctor during the pregnancy. They should note down questions as they think about them, before they are forgotten.

It is important to have confidence in the doctor and, if a change must be made, it should be done early in the pregnancy. To avoid any confusion with medical coverage, it is advisable to notify the British Columbia Medical Plan in writing if a change is made.

## The Dentist:

Care of the mouth is especially important during pregnancy. Tooth decay and gum disease are *preventable* by regular cleaning of teeth and cutting down on sugary foods. The family dentist can develop a plan of action to help the expectant mother keep her teeth in good condition.

### Dental Action Plan for the Mother-To-Be

1)  Prior to a planned pregnancy or early in pregnancy, *an appointment should be made with the family dentist.* He should be informed about the pregnancy as he will probably schedule the routine dental work after the fourth month.

2)  *Proper and thorough toothbrushing and flossing needs to be done at least once every 24 hours.*
    It is extremely important to keep teeth absolutely clean. The combination of hormonal changes of pregnancy and the presence of plaque on teeth can cause gingivitis (red, swollen, bleeding gums). However, regardless of these hormonal changes, if the teeth are clean, the gums will continue to be healthy. The dentist may give additional suggestions about the use of gum stimulators, correct toothbrushing, and floss methods and materials.

3)  *An adequate diet must be maintained.* To ensure healthy teeth and bones for the new baby, the mother needs calcium, phosphorous, protein, and vitamins A, B and D. All are abundant in a healthy diet. Adequate calcium is required early and continuously as the baby's new teeth begin to form in the sixth week of pregnancy. Malnutrition, some diseases and fevers, infections, and use of certain antibiotics (tetracyclines) may cause the developing teeth to become stained, misshaped or imperfect. Because sugars, particularly sucrose, may damage the mother's own teeth, it is a good idea to cut down on them. Further information on nutrition is found in Chapter III.

## The Health Unit:

The local health unit provides a number of services to promote good health during and following pregnancy, and to assist parents in caring for the new baby.

### Prenatal Classes

Prenatal classes are given by public health nurses who are sometimes assisted by nutritionists, physiotherapists, physicians and hospital nurses. Most health units offer early bird classes for parents in the first three months of pregnancy, followed by a series in the last three months. Topics in first classes usually include changes during pregnancy early development of the baby, nutrition and preliminary exercises; the later classes include preparation for labor and delivery, exercises and breathing techniques, care of and feeding the baby, parenting and family relationships. Some health units offer additional classes on topics such as breast-feeding, the single mother, the working mother and caesarian birth.

Expectant parents can either phone or visit their local health unit to register for classes. The numbers are listed on the inside cover of this book.

### Postnatal Groups

Most health units offer postnatal group discussions that cover such topics as adapting lifestyles to the needs of the new baby, infant care and feeding, family planning, and exercises to help the mother regain her figure. This opportunity for parents to receive health information, exchange ideas and receive mutual support is also a pleasant outing for babies and parents.

### Home Visits

Individual prenatal counselling is available if requested. After the baby is born, the liaison nurse from the health unit usually visits new mothers in hospital to explain the available services and help arrange for the return home.

Once home, the new parents can look forward to a visit from the public health nurse within the first two weeks. Unnecessary worry can be avoided by discussing concerns and questions as they arise. Parents requiring assistance or an early visit should contact the health unit. Sometimes the public health nurse who tries to visit is unable to locate a family because they have moved. It is advisable to notify the health unit about any change in address.

### Child Health Conferences — (Well Baby Clinics)

At child health conferences the public health nurses provide information on topics such as breast-feeding, the baby's growth and development, child behavior and nutrition. The conferences also provide an opportunity for the parents to discuss their concerns about their own health or the baby's. Immunization is also available. Further information about the time and location of the closest child health conference may be obtained from the local health unit.

## The Hospital:

Services provided by the community hospital vary according to its size, location and staff.

Prenatally, parents may be referred to the hospital for laboratory or diagnostic tests and in most areas hospital personnel collaborate with the health unit staff in teaching prenatal and postnatal classes.

The care provided by the hospital staff is of particular importance in helping parents throughout the birth process and providing support to the family. The physiotherapist, dietitian, nurse and physician are all members of the basic hospital team; other personnel may be involved, including the pharmacist and social worker. The in-hospital program for care of the mother and baby requires joint participation of the hospital team with the parents and family.

At the end of Chapter 5 information is available about British Columbia hospitals which have been designated as regional referral centres with extra resources for mothers and babies with special needs.

## Other Services:

In some areas of the province other organizations offer prenatal, postnatal and special interest programs. Information about these services may be obtained from the health unit, physician, or the maternity unit of the local hospital. Inquiries about special programs for single mothers may be made at the nearest Human Resources office and the health unit.

A directory of community resources for expectant and new parents has been included on the inside of the front cover of this book.

## NOTES

CHAPTER 2

## UNDERSTANDING PREGNANCY

## Human Reproduction:

Most parents will have learned about the male and female reproductive organs; however, a review is included in this chapter to help them appreciate the changes that take place during pregnancy.

The information also may be helpful to parents when discussing human reproduction with their young children.

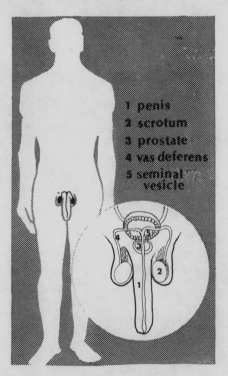

1 penis
2 scrotum
3 prostate
4 vas deferens
5 seminal vesicle

The male reproductive organs are the penis, scrotum, prostate gland, the vas deferens or sperm duct and the seminal vesicle, as illustrated. Inside the scrotum are two testicles which produce the sperm, or male cells of reproduction. A sperm, looking and acting a bit like a tadpole, is microscopic in size. The sperm travel through the vas deferens to a storage pouch, the seminal vesicle. En route they pass the prostate gland which provides a liquid in which the sperm are carried. During ejaculation the millions of sperm travel through the penis into the woman's vagina.

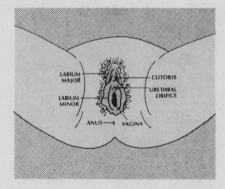

The external part of the female reproductive system is called the vulva, composed of the clitoris, labia majora and labia minora. The clitoris is a small organ hooded by a loose fold of skin. It is located just above the opening (urethra) where the urine passes and is very sensitive to sexual stimulation. The labia majora are large outer folds of skin covering the labia minora, which are smaller, more sensitive folds around the opening to the vagina, which leads to the inside of the body.

The internal reproductive organs are the vagina (birth canal), uterus (womb), ovaries, and Fallopian tubes.

The Fallopian tubes, attached to the uterus, extend trumpet-shaped openings toward the ovaries but are not connected to the ovaries.

After puberty, approximately once a month the ovaries release an ovum (the female cell of reproduction). The ovum or egg travels down the Fallopian tube and if fertilization does not take place, the menstrual flow occurs in approximately two weeks.

If a sperm joins the ovum in the Fallopian tube, fertilization (conception) occurs. In about three days the fertilized ovum reaches the uterus where it becomes attached to the lining and is called an embryo.

The placenta (afterbirth) forms between the embryo and lining of the uterus. The umbilical cord connects the embryo to the placenta to transport nourishment from the mother to the embryo and also carries wastes from the embryo to the mother's bloodstream via the placenta.

After the embryo has grown for eight weeks it is called a fetus. The fetus continues to grow for the next thirty-two weeks until it is delivered as a full-term baby. During that time there are many changes that occur in both the mother and baby as described in the following pages.

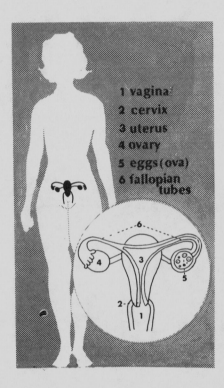

1 vagina
2 cervix
3 uterus
4 ovary
5 eggs (ova)
6 fallopian tubes

The uterus is a pear-shaped, hollow, muscular organ located in the lower abdomen. Its walls are covered with a mucous lining. The neck of the uterus is called the cervix. The cervix opens during labor so that the baby can pass out of the uterus.

Two ovaries are located in the lower abdomen on either side of the uterus.

## Genetic Inheritance:

### Chromosomes

Each human body cell, except reproductive cells (eggs and sperm), contains 46 chromosomes, made up of 23 pairs.

**Diagram 1**

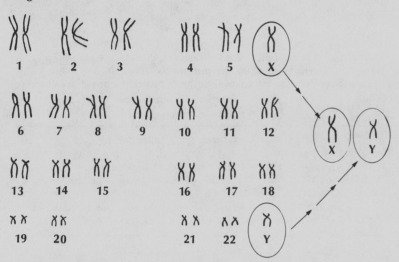

Obviously, if the egg and sperm also contained 46 chromosomes then a fetus resulting from the union of these cells would contain 92 chromosomes. This is not possible and so to ensure that human beings possess the normal human number of chromosomes, a division takes place in formation of the egg or sperm. During this division members of the chromosome pairs separate — each member of a pair going into a different cell.

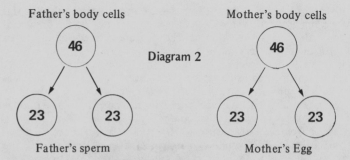

Father's body cells     Mother's body cells

**Diagram 2**

Father's sperm     Mother's Egg

In this way, at the time of conception (fertilization), the father's sperm and mother's egg each contribute half the total number of chromosomes to the unborn child.

**Diagram 3**

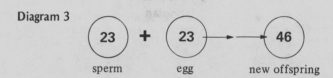

sperm    egg    new offspring

Of the 23 pairs of chromosomes in body cells, 22 of the pairs are alike in both sexes. One pair is different in males and females and this is the pair of chromosomes (sex chromosomes) which is responsible for sex determination. A woman has two X chromosomes in this pair. A man has one X chromosome and one Y chromosome which is much smaller and looks quite different than the X chromosome.

Obviously when the pairs of chromosomes separate to make eggs, a woman will always contribute an X chromosome to the eggs. However, when the pair of sex chromosomes separate in a man to produce sperm, on the average, half the sperm will have an X and half the sperm will have a Y. This means that if a sperm carrying a Y ferilizes the egg then a boy will result as this developing embryo will have an X and a Y as the pair of sex chromosomes. If, however, the sperm which fertilizes the egg is carrying an X then a daughter will result as this developing embryo will have two X's (XX).

This is the normal human situation. It seems, however, that the older a woman gets the more likely it is that mistakes are made in the neat division of her 46 chromosomes into eggs bearing 23. For this reason, women of 38 years and up, who are at this increased risk of having a child with a chromosome disorder, are offered amniocentesis in this province. A very small amount of the fluid in the womb surrounding the fetus is removed during amniocentesis, which is done at the 15th — 16th week of gestation. Floating in this fluid are cells which have originated from the baby. The chromosome makeup of these cells is examined. Any change from the normal human number of 46 can be detected. The most common chromosome abnormality is Down's syndrome (mongolism) which occurs about once in every 600-700 births in B.C., but much more often in older mothers. For that reason, if it is acceptable to a couple and they wish to have pre-natal screening done, amniocentesis is available for them if the mother is over 38 years of age. This age limitation may be changed in the future.

## Genes

Since chromosomes are paired, each segment in one chromosome has a corresponding segment in its partner. Genes consist of small segments of chromosomes which control specific hereditary characteristics. There are thousands of genes distributed along the chromosome. It follows that genes, as they are specific parts of the chromosomes, are paired. For a particular gene pair, an individual will have inherited one member of the gene pair from the mother (because one of the chromosomes of the pair came from the mother) and one of the genes of the pair from the father (because the other chromosome in the pair came from him).

When a particular gene is considered, an individual may have a double dose of the exact same form of that gene or may have two different forms of the gene (two different alleles). Alleles (alternative forms of a gene) may be dominant or recessive. A recessive allele is one that has to be present in an individual in a double dose before its effect is seen. A dominant allele is one whose effect is seen even if only one of the pair of genes is of this type.

From a practical point of view there are four patterns of inheritance of genetic disorders that are important in human beings.

The first of these four patterns is autosomal dominant inheritance. In this mode of inheritance an affected parent has one dose of the dominant form of the gene and because it is dominant, is affected with a particular disorder. Obviously, when the parent's gene pair separates in going into the eggs or the sperm, approximately half of these will have the dominant gene which causes the particular disorder. There are about 600 different disorders caused by dominant genes. Some of these are things like Huntington's chorea, neurofibromatosis, and Marfan's syndrome. The diagram below shows how in autosomal dominant inheritance half the offspring are affected.

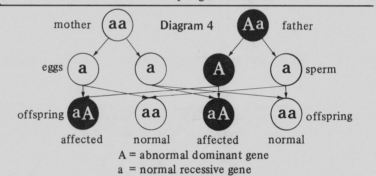

A = abnormal dominant gene
a = normal recessive gene

The second type of single gene inheritance we are concerned with is autosomal recessive inheritance, in which the parents themselves are completely normal but each of them is carrying one dose of a recessive gene. The only time that this will cause a problem is when an individual receives a double dose of it. The diagram below shows how two people who are carriers of the same recessive gene have a one in four chance of a child being affected with the recessive disorder.

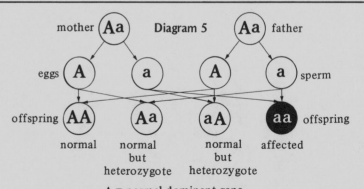

A = normal dominant gene
a = abnormal recessive gene

In the last two types of inherited disorders, a gene is linked to the X chromosome, and those which are multi-factorial or due to several gene pairs. It is not possible in a book of this size to go into these in detail. If any couple has a family history of a particular disorder, it is wise (and often reassuring) to ask their family doctor for a referral for genetic counselling. This is available in this province at the genetics counselling clinic run by the Department of Medical Genetics, University of British Columbia.

Any couple who have had one child with some type of congenital malformation deserve to have counselling with regard to the likelihood for this to happen again. In an increasing number of conditions there are also ways of very early detecting if the next pregnancy is affected. Many people, once they have had a child with a problem, think that their risk is much higher than it may be. Usually, couples find a thorough discussion of possible treatment or prevention very helpful in relieving their anxieties. Most people are justified in expecting that if they themselves are normal and have a normal pregnancy they are guaranteed a normal baby. However, it should be remembered that 2-3% of all babies have some congenital abnormality. By congenital abnormality is meant simply some problem which can be detected at birth. Some of these are genetic in origin, some are not. With the increasing number of seriously handicapping conditions that can be detected early in pregnancy, and the simplicity of estimating risk, it makes sense that any couple concerned about their family background should seek competent counselling.

### Twinning

There are two kinds of twins; identical and fraternal. Identical twins result from a single fertilized egg which splits into two individuals at a very early stage of development. It follows necessarily that these twins are always of the same sex and, because they have identical genetic constitutions, will be very similar in appearance and, on testing for any genetic traits, such as blood groups, they will be the same. Fraternal twins occur when two eggs shed in the same menstrual cycle, are fertilized separately. These twins are really only as similar as any other siblings. They are twins because they are carried in the womb at the same time. If there is a history in the mother's family of fraternal twinning she has more than the usual chance of producing twins. The incidence of twinning is 1 in 86 births. In future pregnancies, a mother who has produced one set of fraternal twins has a 3%

chance of recurrence. Fraternal twins occur about twice as often as identical twins.

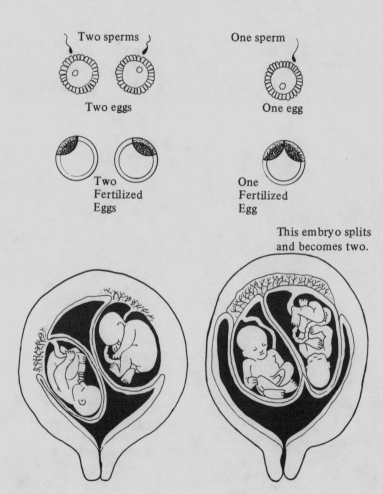

FRATERNAL TWINS     IDENTICAL TWINS

Two sperms        One sperm

Two eggs        One egg

Two Fertilized Eggs        One Fertilized Egg

This embryo splits and becomes two.

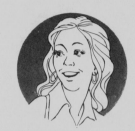

Physical Changes that Usually Occur in the Mother During Pregnancy:

| APPROXIMATE TIME/WEEKS | WHAT'S HAPPENING | MOTHER NEEDS TO |
|---|---|---|
| First Trimester | *Amenorrhea* (absence of menstruation) | |
| 1-4 | Hormone changes occur, stopping the menstrual cycle so that the uterine wall lining will build up to cushion and feed baby. | - eat a variety of foods from each of the four food groups daily (see page 24). |
| | *Breasts Tingling and Tense* | |
| 5 | Hormones cause changes in breast tissues to prepare for nursing. | |
| | *Fatigue* | |
| | Energy needs of pregnancy are greater than before. Mother tires much more easily. | - allow for extra rest; - learn limitations, stopping short of fatigue; - alternate periods of activity and rest. |
| | *Nausea* ("Morning Sickness") | |
| 6 | Caused by hormonal action, tension and/or fatigue. Usually lasts about 8-12 weeks only but may persist longer in the tense, nervous, apprehensive mother. Can occur anytime of day. | - eat smaller more frequent meals; - avoid drinking liquids with meals until nausea passes; - a dry cracker in the morning before getting up may help. |
| | *Frequency of Urination* | |
| | Uterus is pressing on bladder, decreasing its capacity. The increased production of estrogen and progesterone is responsible for increased circulation to the pelvic area, including the bladder. | - restrict amount of fluids taken in the evening. |

| APPROXIMATE TIME/WEEKS | WHAT'S HAPPENING | MOTHER NEEDS TO |
|---|---|---|
| | *Increased Vaginal Secretions* (thin and milky) | |
| | Due to hormones (again) and increased congestion. | - keep area clean and dry. |
| | *Introspective and Sleepy* | |
| | Thought to be hormonal. Part of natural protection for mother and baby; mother doesn't feel overactive. | - realize that this is normal and need not be fought; <br> - take it easy! |
| | *Breasts Enlarged* <br> *Areola Around Nipples Darkens* | |
| | Continued changes in breast tissues in preparation for breast feeding. | - wear a good supporting bra for comfort; <br> - wear a light bra for sleeping if breasts are really heavy. |
| | *Lightheadedness* | |
| 6-9 | The circulatory system is working harder and may adapt slowly to standing or sitting. | - get up or change positions slowly; <br> - maintain good posture; to do exercises regularly; <br> - avoid skipping meals. |
| | *Shortness of Breath* | |
| | Control of body chemistry changes, requiring increased breathing. | - realize that this is normal. |
| | *Montgomery's Tubercles on* <br> *Areola of Breasts* | |
| 12th week or after | These are small lumps containing fatty substances which lubricate areola of breast. | - know these changes are normal. |
| | *Chloasma (Mask of Pregnancy)* <br> *and Linea Nigra Darkens* | |
| | Brownish "tan" on face and line running from the navel to the pubic area. | - know that these signs will occur in some women and that the mask disappears after the baby is born; the linea nigra may remain. |

| APPROXIMATE TIME/WEEKS | WHAT'S HAPPENING | MOTHER NEEDS TO |
|---|---|---|
| Second Trimester | *Little Nausea, Less Bladder Pressure, Less Tired* | |
| | Uterus rising up in abdomen — takes pressure off pelvic organs. Body more adjusted to state of pregnancy. | - be aware that the dangers of miscarriage or spontaneous abortion are mainly over;<br>- enjoy her pregnancy;<br>- increase diet nutrients, see page 24 . |
| | *Colostrum (May Begin Anytime From Now Until Birth)* | |
| 16th week | This water-protein matter is the prelude to breast milk. | - not worry about ability to nurse if colostrum not present; see page 36 on breast changes and care. |
| | *Quickening* | |
| 18-22 | Movement of baby felt by mother. May occur earlier, or later than noted here. | - note the date, and tell the doctor on the next visit. This is a useful milestone by which to date the expected birth. |
| | *Low Back Pain* | |
| 20-21 or after | Due to stretching of ligaments attached to uterus. Increase in size of abdomen causing curvature of spine. Normal softening of pelvic joints. May also be due to poor posture. | - maintain good posture, see page 28;<br>- wear supportive shoes, see page 33;<br>- wear a non-constricting girdle if needed. |
| | *Throbbing of Legs* | |
| | Pressure in abdomen sometimes causing pooling of blood in leg veins. Those women with a tendency of varicose veins may find them worse during pregnancy. | - elevate legs when sitting or reclining permits;<br>- wear support stockings if recommended ("Knee Highs" and garters should not be worn as they constrict circulation). |
| | *Constipation (Hard, Dry, Bowel Movements)* | |
| | Early in pregnancy as a result of changing food habits or hormone action that slows bowel activity; later it may be caused by enlargement | - drink plenty of fluids;<br>- increase roughage and fibrous food in diet;<br>- exercise regularly — walking, swimming, etc.; |

| APPROXIMATE TIME/WEEKS | WHAT'S HAPPENING | MOTHER NEEDS TO |
|---|---|---|
| | of the uterus, which displaces the intestines and compresses the colon. | - put feet upon a foot stool when using toilet; so that the thighs provide support and comfort for the abdomen;<br>- take laxatives only as selected by the doctor. |
| | *Weight Begins to Increase Rapidly (3-4 Pounds per Month) Baby Can be Felt* | |
| 24 | Rapid growth in size of baby from this time on. Physical changes in placenta and increase in body fluid. | - to maintain good posture and body mechanics and good nutrition.  See pages 24, 28. |
| Third Trimester | *Striae (Purple or Red Marks) on Abdomen and Breast* | |
| 30 weeks and later | Due to stretching of the skin and increased activity of hormones from the adrenal cortex. | - massage skin with lotion or oil to alleviate the itching. |
| | *Fatigue Increases* | |
| | Due to new demands by both the fetus and the mother's body. | - eat an adequate diet;<br>- have frequent rest periods;<br>- know personal limitations;<br>- rest *before* getting tired. |
| | *Braxton-Hicks Contractions Painless Uterine Contractions May be Felt* | |
| | Irregular contractions of the uterus, become noticeable now. | - use breathing exercises;<br>- tell the doctor if the contractions are particularly painful. |
| | *Muscle Cramps in Legs, Especially at Night* | |
| | Thought to be due to pressure on abdominal nerves, fatigue and calcium-phosphorus imbalance. | - maintain good posture;<br>- avoid fatigue;<br>- elevate the feet; |

| APPROXIMATE TIME/WEEKS | WHAT'S HAPPENING | MOTHER NEEDS TO |
|---|---|---|

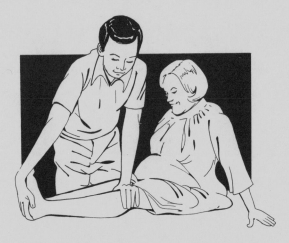

- *tell the doctor* as he may want to prescribe extra calcium or other medicine to correct the imbalance;
- press foot against a firm surface to relieve foot cramps;
- straighten leg and have someone push back on knee when lying down, and press sole of foot against hand, keep leg straight and toes pointing up.

*Fatigue and Some Depression*

35    Feelings of awkwardness and impatience at seemingly endlessness of pregnancy. Frustration with inability to keep up with pre-pregnancy activities to some degree.

- *remember* it will not be long before the baby is born.
- talk things over with a friend, especially one who's had a baby and understands.

*Heartburn and Flatulence*
*Constipation, Frequent Voiding,*

36    Due to pressure of uterus on stomach, bladder, and intestines, and hormonal action.

- eat small, frequent meals;
- drink liquids between meals, not with them;
- avoid highly spiced and fried foods;
- *Not Take Baking Soda;*
- prevent constipation — see page 68;
- have regular bowel habits;
- discuss relief for hemorrhoids with doctor.

*Hemorrhoids*

Due to pressure interfering with circulation in the veins; aggravated by constipation.

- see page 69.

| APPROXIMATE TIME/WEEKS | WHAT'S HAPPENING | MOTHER NEEDS TO |
|---|---|---|
| | *Shortness of Breath* | |
| | Top of uterus pressing against diaphragm (lung capacity is decreased). Most troublesome when attempting to lie down. | - elevate head of bed or prop head up with several pillows to assume a semi-sitting position for sleeping. |
| | *Breathing Easier — Decreased Abdominal Distention* | |
| 37-38 | With first pregnancy "lightening" has occurred. Feels like baby dropped! Uterus settles down in pelvic cavity. With subsequent pregnancies lightening may not occur until labor starts. | - tell doctor that this has happened. |
| | *Frequency of Urination* | |
| | Uterus again pressing on bladder decreasing its capacity. | - do exercises as instructed. |
| | *Weight Loss 2-3 Pounds Increase in (False Labor) Contractions, a Burst of Energy Less Movement of Baby* | |
| 3 to 4 days before labor | Due to changes in placental function. | |
| | Mother feels more aware of changes occurring. Baby is getting ready. | - not become involved in strenuous activities; - conserve energy! - complete packing for hospital and last minute household arrangements. |

THE GREAT DAY IS APPROACHING!

## Emotional Changes During Pregnancy:

Pregnancy is an altered state of the body, bringing many changes in the body systems. There are also emotional changes. An expectant mother may experience sudden and unexplained mood changes and bouts of crying or laughing. She also may feel very irritable and self-centered at times. Thoughts and fantasies may come to mind that have never been entertained previously.

Her feelings about the pregnancy itself also vary between a sense of elation or well being and alternatively, not enjoying the pregnancy

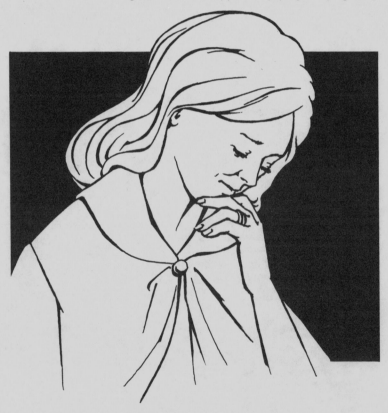

at all. At times, the expectant mother may need extra attention and affection and feel very dependent upon others.

*Varying Moods Should Not Be Alarming!* They are experienced by most expectant mothers and are caused by the many hormonal changes going on in the body. They are also part of the mental task of preparing for parenthood. It is helpful to realize that these moods are normal and temporary, although knowing this does not reduce them.

It is well for the expectant parents to realize that both partners have emotional reactions. The father may feel jealous of the mother's ability to carry the baby, insecure about his ability to be a father, or guilt and helplessness about his wife's emotional ups and downs.

Open discussion of feelings can clarify misunderstandings and prevent unwarranted fears. Myths, fears and emotional concerns should be freely discussed with the doctor or public health nurse. Talking about feelings and concerns can foster a healthy marital relationship, and is of particular importance if changes need to be made in sexual relationships.

## Sexual Relations During Pregnancy:

Many couples are reluctant to discuss sexual relations during pregnancy with the physician and/or nurse, and all too often the professional team does not provide an opportunity for discussion of this important topic. Misinformation and many myths exist regarding whether or not to continue sexual intercourse during pregnancy. Does it hurt the baby? Will it cause miscarriage? Will "the bag of waters" burst?

These and many other questions may come to mind during pregnancy. Sexual relationships during pregnancy will be largely dependant upon the relationship before pregnancy, the partners' attitudes to the pregnancy and their concerns about it. In a recent review of reports, four patterns of sexual functioning were found to emerge and are shown in the graphs on page 17. These graphs show that some couples experienced a steady increase in sexual intercourse throughout the three trimesters. Other couples experienced a decrease in the first and third trimesters and an increase in the second. Some couples had

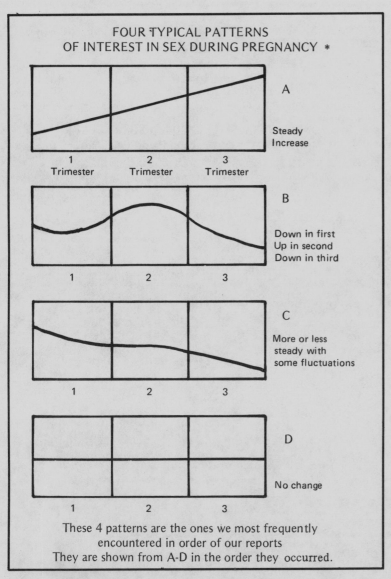

## FOUR TYPICAL PATTERNS
## OF INTEREST IN SEX DURING PREGNANCY *

A

Steady
Increase

1
Trimester     2
Trimester     3
Trimester

B

Down in first
Up in second
Down in third

1     2     3

C

More or less
steady with
some fluctuations

1     2     3

D

No change

1     2     3

These 4 patterns are the ones we most frequently
encountered in order of our reports
They are shown from A-D in the order they occurred.

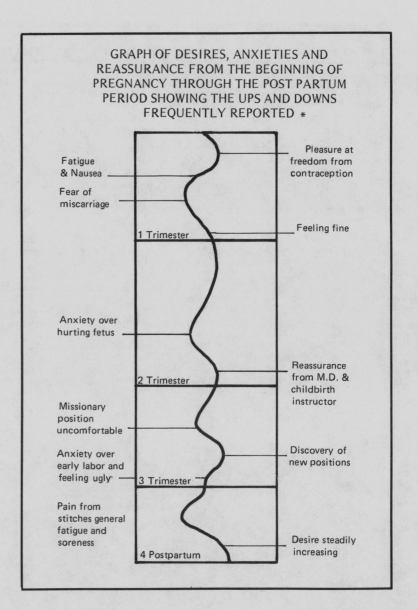

## GRAPH OF DESIRES, ANXIETIES AND
## REASSURANCE FROM THE BEGINNING OF
## PREGNANCY THROUGH THE POST PARTUM
## PERIOD SHOWING THE UPS AND DOWNS
## FREQUENTLY REPORTED *

Fatigue
& Nausea

Fear of
miscarriage

Pleasure at
freedom from
contraception

1 Trimester

Feeling fine

Anxiety over
hurting fetus

2 Trimester

Reassurance
from M.D. &
childbirth
instructor

Missionary
position
uncomfortable

Anxiety over
early labor and
feeling ugly

Discovery of
new positions

3 Trimester

Pain from
stitches general
fatigue and
soreness

4 Postpartum

Desire steadily
increasing

*E. Bing and L. Colman, *Making Love During Pregnancy*, New York,
Bantam Books Inc., 1977, pp. 48-49.

a steady pattern of less intercourse as the pregnancy advanced while others showed no change.

The graphs show why couples decreased or increased intercourse and the reasons for the changes. A decrease in intercourse may occur for some due to fatigue and nausea in the first three months, whereas other couples may find greater pleasure due to increased freedom from contraception at this time.

As pregnancy advances, changes in positions may be necessary and experimenting with different techniques such as lying side by side, sitting, or approaching from the rear may help to find more comfortable and acceptable positions.

Frequently the father may lack the desire for intercourse for a short interval during the last trimester and the mother may feel dismay or hurt at this rejection if she does not realize that this is a normal and temporary situation.

Generally, sexual intercourse or sex play can continue during pregnancy. If there is vaginal bleeding, pain or loss of fluid from the uterus, the doctor should be told as soon as possible so that he can give specific instructions and possibly alternate avenues of sexual relations may be explored. A tender, intimate loving relationship helps in adjusting to the emotional aspects associated with pregnancy and helps the partners adapt to parenthood when lovemaking goes beyond caring for each other and spreads to embrace the family unit.[1]

[1]E. Bing and L. Colman, *Making Love During Pregnancy*. New York, Bantam Books. 1977, p. 159.

## NOTES

## Growth and Development of the Fetus:

The development of the baby from two tiny egg cells is truly a remarkable story. Some of the main events in development are included in the following chart.

| TIME | ACTUAL SIZE | DESCRIPTION |
|---|---|---|

1st Trimester

1 day — Fertilization – union of sperm and ovum.

7 days — 0.3 mm — Fertilized egg (ovum) becomes implanted in lining of uterus. Afterbirth (placenta) begins to develop.

2 weeks — A layered disc on uterus wall. Mother has missed her first menstrual cycle.

4 weeks — Head is 1/3 size of entire embryo — rudiments of eyes, ears, nose, spine, digestive tract and nervous system are formed. Tube for future heart starts beating.

8 weeks — 1 gm (1/3 oz.) — All systems and organs present that will be found in full term baby. Now called a *fetus*. Heart is functioning.

12 weeks (3 months) — 15 gm-30 gm (½ oz.-1 oz.) — Sex can be distinguished, "baby" teeth buds present. Rudimentary kidneys secrete urine to bladder. Can move in amniotic fluid (bag of water), but cannot be felt by the mother.

The first trimester (first three months) is a crucial time in the life of the baby (fetus) because such rapid growth and development occur. *GOOD MATERNAL NUTRITION IS VITAL.* At this time, the baby is susceptible to the environmental dangers of smoking, infections, drugs and x-rays. This is why advice about health care should be sought early.

**Second Trimester**

TIME & SIZE

DESCRIPTION

3rd to 6th month

Actual
Size At
About 4
months
weight =
approx.
120 gm
(4 oz.)

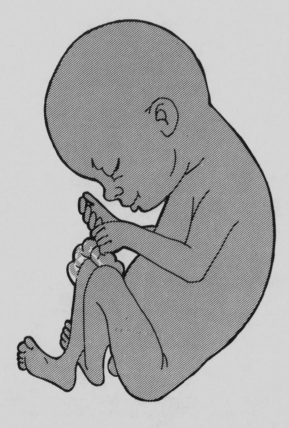

1)  Fetus grows an average of 1.5 mm per day.

2)  Gains approximately 1000 gm (2-3 lbs.).

3)  Fetal heart can first be heard with a stethescope between 18th to 28th week.

4)  A fine downy hair (lanugo) appears all over the body but may be present at full-term.

5)  222 bones are formed and calcium is utilized from mother's circulation — hence the need for foods containing calcium.

6)  The skin is thin, shiny and covered with a creamy protective coating called vernix.

7)  Baby may suck thumb!

The second trimester is crucial for refinement of the physical characteristics of the fetus. The major brain development is from now until 18 months after birth. The fetus cannot live outside the mother's body because the respiratory and cardiovascular systems are not adequately developed.

20

### Third Trimester

| TIME & SIZE | | DESCRIPTION |
|---|---|---|

7th to 9th month

Average Weight at Birth:

- for girls 3,280 gm (7 lbs.)

- for boys 3,410 gm (7½ lbs.)


Average Height: 58 cm (20")

Fetus gains about 2,500 gm (5 lbs.) in these three months, and grows 23 cm (8").

The skin smooths as the fat forms under it.

Baby can survive if delivered before full-term but needs special care. The closer birth is to full-term the more ready the baby is to cope with the birth process and to exchange the shelter of the uterus for life in the outside world.

---

## Every Pregnancy is Unique:

Every expectant parent should recognize that no two pregnancies are alike. After all, it is a different time in the parent's life and the developing fetus has his or her own set of characteristics.

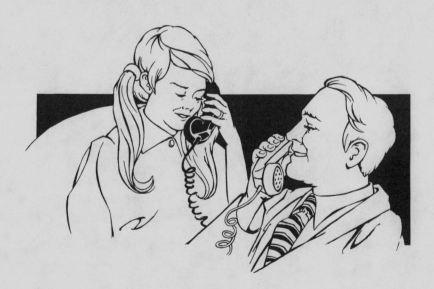

Parents have their own unique physical and emotional makeup and therefore should expect their experience to be different compared with their friends'. Thanks to scientific knowledge, doctors and hospital personnel have the ability and equipment available to give excellent care and to deal with difficulties that may be encountered during pregnancy, labor and delivery.

Because of advancing scientific knowledge, frequently difficulties can be anticipated and appropriate care taken in advance of the baby's birth. It is important for the expectant parents to recognize and report elements of risk to the doctor. The following list includes items that should be reported.

1. Any illness with or without fever. (Do not take any medication, even those purchased without a prescription, unless ordered by the doctor.)

2. Any elevation in body temperature.

3. Any exposure to rubella (German Measles).

4. Rashes of any kind.

5. Itching of the skin.

6.  Excessive fatigue.

7.  Dizziness, headaches, dimness or blurring of vision.

8.  Swelling of feet, hands or face.

9.  Sudden weight gain.

10. Frequent vomiting.

11. Abdominal pain.

12. Bleeding from the vagina, bowel or bladder.

13. A burning feeling associated with urinating.

14. Colored, frothy, foul-smelling vaginal discharge or one causing local itchiness.

15. Gush or trickle of water from the vagina.

16. Concern about persistant negative feelings about the pregnancy and care of the baby.

17. Periods of weeping or depression that don't go away.

18. Concern about medical conditions in the family such as hereditary diseases, diabetes, high blood pressure and kidney disease.

**NOTES**

CHAPTER 3

# EFFECTS OF LIFESTYLE ON PREGNANCY

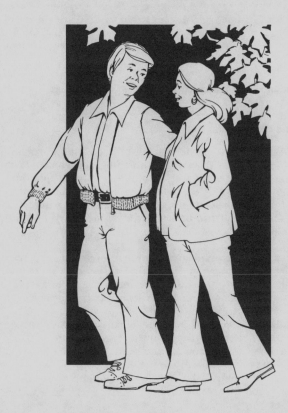

At conception, the baby inherited genes that will determine the physical, emotional, and mental characteristics with which to face life, but for the first nine months the baby's growth and development may be altered by the mother's lifestyle and environment.

Using the following list, an expectant mother can look at her lifestyle and identify factors that should be changed because they pose a risk to the baby's development.

## PRENATAL LIFESTYLE RISKS
(Check with pages as indicated below)

| Cause of Risk | Page No. | Risk Present | | Comments |
|---|---|---|---|---|
| | | Yes | No | |
| 1) Inadequate Diet | 23 | | | |
| 2) Poor Weight Gain | 25 | | | |
| 3) Excessive Alcohol Intake | 30 | | | |
| 4) Misuse of Drugs | 29 | | | |
| 5) Smoking Cigarettes | 28 | | | |
| 6) Poor Health | 30 | | | |
| 7) Emotional Stress | 31 | | | |

It is hoped that information in the following pages will help the expectant mother to understand and reduce the lifestyle risks to her baby. There are of course other factors such as inadequate income, poor obstetrical history, medical problems, and mother's age (under 18 or over 40) that should be discussed with the doctor or public health nurse.

## Nutrition:

A woman's diet during pregnancy is important to both mother and baby. As the mother's body is the baby's first environment, the quality and quantity of food eaten during pregnancy affects the baby's lifetime health and achievement. The developing fetus is not the only individual affected by a pregnant woman's diet. The mother benefits from a healthy pregnancy and the knowledge that she is providing the best materials and environment possible.

A wise approach to healthful eating during pregnancy is to establish good eating habits before conception and to continue these habits during pregnancy and breast-feeding. A woman's caloric and nutrient needs increase throughout pregnancy as the fetus grows. Particular attention should be given to increased requirements for seven nutrients:

Protein
Iron
Calcium
Folic Acid
Vitamin A
Vitamin C
Vitamin D

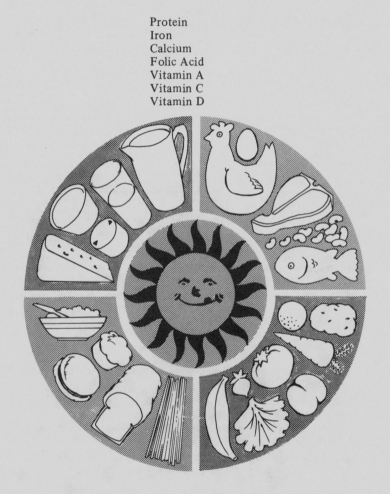

## Canada's Food Guide for the Pregnant Woman

Canada's Food Guide recommends that Canadians eat a variety of foods from each group every day. The Four Food Groups and their recommended number of daily servings for a pregnant woman are:

| | |
|---|---|
| Milk and Milk Products | 4 servings |
| Meat and Alternates | 2 servings |
| Fruits and Vegetables | 4-5 servings |
| Bread and Cereals | 3-5 servings |

Foods selected according to Canada's Food Guide can supply 1000-1400 calories daily. The average, non-pregnant woman of child-bearing age with a characteristic activity pattern requires approximately 1900-2100 calories daily. The additional energy requirements over those supplied by following Canada's Food Guide are obtained by increasing the number and size of servings from the Four Food Groups or by adding other foods.

Calories must be increased above normal levels during pregnancy to provide energy and material for fetal and maternal growth. The average woman requires an extra 100 calories daily during the first trimester (first three months), and an extra 300 calories daily during the second and third trimesters. An example of 100 calories is a glass of 2% milk or a piece of buttered bread. An example of 300 calories is a cheese, meat or peanut butter sandwich; or a large glass of milk with a bran muffin and an orange. A very active woman, or a woman who is underweight will require a greater increase in calories. These women should consult the nutritionist, public health nurse or physician for additional information.

Pregnancy is *NOT* a time to lose weight and calories should never be restricted. Those women concerned about gaining more than the recommended 25 pounds, or who are gaining too quickly should choose foods that contain the nutrients known to be essential to the health of both mother and fetus and which do not contain excessive calories.

It doesn't matter whether foods are eaten in three large meals, five smaller ones, or a combination of meals and snacks. It is essential that meals and snacks be made up of foods supplying body building nutrients, not just fats and sugars. For example, potato chips, pastries and other sweets offer many calories with very few nutrients. As well, these foods are filling and leave a person with less of an appetite for foods that are really necessary.

A total weight gain of approximately 25 pounds is advisable during pregnancy for a healthy woman who was not underweight before pregnancy. When twins are expected the suggested total weight gain increases to approximately 35 pounds. The following table outlines the components of weight gain during a normal pregnancy with a single infant.

| COMPONENTS OF WEIGHT GAIN DURING PREGNANCY (AVERAGE) | | |
|---|---|---|
| Component | Pounds | Kilograms* |
| Baby | 7.5 | 3.4 |
| Placenta | 1.5 | 0.6 |
| Aminotic Fluid | 2.0 | 1.0 |
| Uterine Size Increase | 2.0 | 1.0 |
| Breast Size Increase | 1.0 | 0.4 |
| Blood Volume Increase | 3.3 | 1.5 |
| Increase in fluid between cells | 3.3 | 1.5 |
| Mother's stored reserves | 4.5 | 2.0 |
| TOTAL | 25.1 | 11.4 |

* 1 kilogram is equal to 2.2 pounds

The *rate* of weight gained during pregnancy is also important. The weight gain should be slow during the first trimester and more rapid, but steady, during the last six months. The following graph illustrates a normal pattern of weight gain during pregnancy.

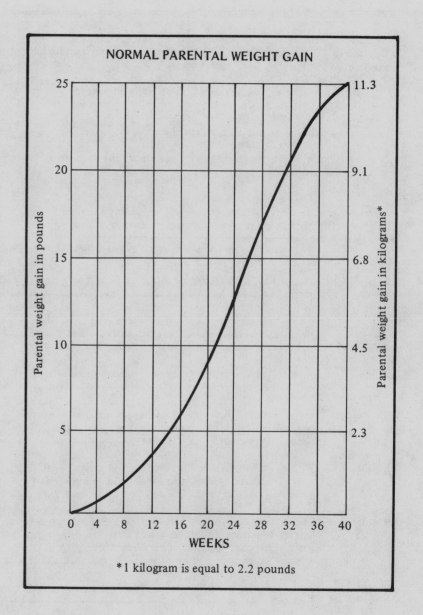

NORMAL PARENTAL WEIGHT GAIN

*1 kilogram is equal to 2.2 pounds

Each pregnant woman should record her weight gain every one to two weeks. The nutritionist, public health nurse or physician should be notified if:

- the pattern of weight gain varies significantly from the pattern shown,

- too much or too little weight is gained, or

- the weight gain is less than 17 pounds by the 30th week of pregnancy.

Weight loss at delivery averages 11 to 13 pounds (baby, fluid, placenta). The total weight gained during pregnancy is usually lost within 6-12 weeks of delivery, particularly if the infant is breast fed.

Pregnant and breast-feeding women require more fluids than a non-pregnant woman. A pregnant woman should try to drink the equivalent of 6-10 glasses of fluid each day. Sources of fluids include milk, juice, water, soup and ice cream.

Some women need additional advice on nutrition during pregnancy. A woman should contact the nutritionist, public health nurse or physician for additional information if any of the risk factors listed in the section on "Effect of Lifestyle on Pregnancy" apply to her.

Additional reading on nutrition in pregnancy is available in the booklet, *Eating For A Baby*. Copies are available from the local health unit.

## GOOD DIETARY SOURCES OF CERTAIN NUTRIENTS

Protein
: Milk, cheese, eggs, meat, fish, poultry, dried legumes (peas, beans, lentils), cereals, nuts, bread, peanut butter.

Iron
: Liver, kidney, red meat, dried fruits, egg yolk, dark green leafy vegetables, whole grain and enriched breads and cereals.

Calcium
: Milk and dairy products, canned sardines and salmon with bones, broccoli, egg yolk, greens.

Folic Acid
: Liver, kidney, brewer's yeast, mushrooms, asparagus, broccoli, lima beans, spinach, orange juice, lemons, bananas, strawberries, cantaloupe.

Vitamin A
: Whole or fortified milk, fortified margarine, butter, eggs, liver and kidney, tomatoes, cantaloupe, dark green vegetables, yellow-fleshed vegetables and fruits.

Vitamin C
: Citrus fruits and juices, vitaminized apple juice, most berries, tomatoes and their juice, cantaloupe, mango, papaya, cabbage, broccoli, cauliflower, brussel sprouts, spinach, green pepper, turnip, white potato.

Vitamin D
: Eggs, fortified milk, butter, fortified margarine, fish liver oils.

## Physical Fitness, Rest, Relaxation:

Balancing the daily activities of work, rest and recreation is just as important for healthful living during pregnancy as it is at any other time. It is wise to get eight hours of sleep at night, to set aside regular times of the day for rest and relaxation, and to alternate periods of activity with periods of rest.

During the latter stages of pregnancy, it may be difficult to sleep and it may be necessary to try pillows in various positions to obtain comfort. Many women find it comfortable to lie on their side with a pillow tucked under the abdomen or waist and one between the knees.

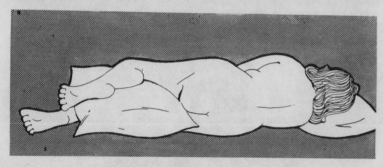

Learning muscle relaxation is as important as sleeping. Sitting down with the feet up several times a day helps. Instructions on how to relax at home and at work are given at prenatal classes.

Most tasks can be done as usual, but as pregnancy progresses, the centre of balance changes and consequently, reaching and climbing should be avoided to prevent falls. Standing should be avoided for activities that can be done in sitting position, but legs should not be crossed while sitting down.

In addition to regular activities, out-of-doors recreation should be enjoyed. Participation in sports depends largely upon the level of activity prior to pregnancy. Anything that can be done well is acceptable unless balance is involved or there is danger of falling. Fatigue comes suddenly during pregnancy so rest periods should be taken before becoming tired. Participation in sports and strenuous

activities should be discussed with the doctor so that a decision can be reached together.

## The Mother-to-be at Work:

Early in pregnancy the subject of how long to continue working should be discussed with the father, employer, and physician and an agreeable plan decided upon. It is usually fine to continue to work if the job is not tiring nor unduly stressful; in fact, it can be good to keep occupied.

A woman with an office job probably does less strenuous work than the average homemaker who is at home all day; however, consideration should be given to swtiching to a less physically demanding or less hazardous occupation if any of the following situations exist:

- heavy physical work;

- long hours;

- lifting or constant standing;

- risk of falling;

- contact with hazardous substances (chemicals, gases, etc.).

Whatever the occupation, two brief rest periods during the day are necessary. Lying down once during a rest period will help. A nutritious meal plus snacks are important during the work period.

A working mother will need to give careful thought and planning to have the extra rest and relaxation required. Perhaps a quiet spot can be found for a coffee (milk) break where the feet can be elevated on a chair or stool.

Maybe a couch or a foam mat can be found to lie down on during the lunch hour. Sometimes it helps if needs are discussed with the employer, as special favours are not being sought, just necessities for the mother and baby.

If standing for long periods is required on the job, it is more comfortable to rest one foot somewhat higher on a ledge, low stool, or even a thick book. This helps to straighten the spine and relieve backache. Swinging one's weight from one foot to the other helps the circulation and prevents fatigue and cramps. Good posture must be practiced. Exercises, such as pulling in the abdomen (as far back as possible), tucking in the buttocks and relaxing the shoulders also help. Sometimes a girdle is needed (see page 33).

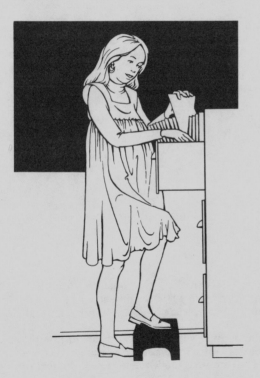

Up-to-date information on maternity benefits is available from Unemployment Insurance, Canada Unemployment Centre, (listed under Government of Canada in the telephone book) early in pregnancy. Sometimes private plans or company policies provide maternity benefits. The British Columbia Maternity Protection Act should be read and is available for 25¢ from the Queen's Printer, Parliament Buildings, Victoria, British Columbia, V8V 1X4.

## Smoking, Drugs, Alcohol and Illness:

### Smoking
During recent years young parents have had information available to help them plan when they will have children. As more and more pregnancies are planned, parents are also becoming aware of the need to change their lifestyles to give the baby the best chance of being healthy.

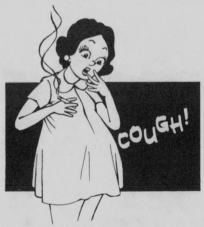

In view of the recent scientific findings about the adverse effects of cigarette smoking (which subjects the fetus to decreased oxygen and to poisons such as cyanide and nicotine) many parents have stopped smoking in preparation for the planned pregnancy. In this way the mother reduces the risk to the baby of being low in birth weight, and a non-smoking father provides a smoke-free environment for the baby after birth.

A mother who is unable to stop smoking during pregnancy should at least cut down as carbon monoxide levels are elevated in both the mother's and fetus' blood and this decreases the oxygen available to the developing baby.

Help is available to anyone wishing to stop smoking from:


- The British Columbia Lung Association
  906 West Broadway
  Vancouver, B.C.
  V5Z 1K7
  Telephone: 731-4961

- Health Education Centre
  3019 Shakespeare
  Victoria, B.C.
  V8R 4H6
  Telephone: 595-4554

  or: P.O. Box 35399, Station E
      Vancouver, B.C.
      V6M 4G5


- Local Tuberculosis, Cancer and/or Health Associations

If these organizations are not available locally contact the health unit for information.


## Drugs

The use of drugs during pregnancy is a complex topic. Since the world-wide publicity which followed the thalidomide experience, most parents are aware that some drugs taken by the mother can cause malformed babies and that drugs known to cause defects should be avoided.

Physicians try to avoid prescribing medication to prevent any unnecessary risk to the developing fetus. Although the likelihood of major malformation is over after the first twelve weeks, every effort is made to AVOID MEDICATIONS during the remaining months of the pregnancy. When drugs are needed, the mother should work with the

doctor to ensure that problem drugs or dangerous combinations are avoided.

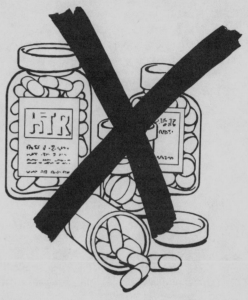

### Key Points to Remember

- *Prescribed* drugs should *not* be discontinued without consulting the doctor.

- Aspirin, cold remedies, and other "over the counter" pills should not be taken unless advised by the doctor.

- Vitamin pills are not a substitute for a healthy diet and any dietary supplement required should be under the doctor's guidance.

- Soft drugs such as marijuana are best avoided.


Narcotics such as heroin and opium can have serious effects on the unborn baby. Mothers who use "street drugs" habitually should let the doctor know and find out how they can give their baby the best chance for a healthy start in life.

In summary:

**NO MEDICATIONS OF ANY KIND SHOULD BE TAKEN EXCEPT ON THE INSTRUCTIONS OF THE PHYSICIAN**

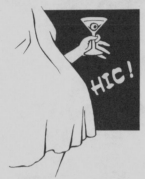

### Alcohol

Alcohol is a drug that passes from the mother to the unborn fetus through the placenta, and thus, when mother drinks, the fetus is exposed to a drug that can delay mental and physical functioning.

There is growing evidence to suggest that pregnant mothers should *not* drink alcoholic beverages at all. The family doctor will want to know about his patient's drinking habits so that the necessary care and additional nutritional counselling may be given. Mothers who have difficulty with problem drinking can receive help from organizations such as the Alcohol and Drug Commission of B.C. or Alcoholics Anonymous.

These services are usually listed in the telephone directory under "Alcohol and Drug Services", but if not found, the health unit can be contacted for the needed information.

Help may also be obtained by writing to:

Alcohol and Drug Commission
307 West Broadway
Vancouver, B.C. V5Y 1P9

### Illness

The growing fetus is completely dependent upon the parents for protection against environmental hazards likely to interfere with normal growth and development. It is wise, therefore, to avoid contact with those who are ill. If illness occurs in the family, the doctor should be informed immediately and medications avoided except as prescribed by the physician.

Communicable diseases, especially German Measles (rubella), should be avoided. The harmful effects of rubella to the unborn baby

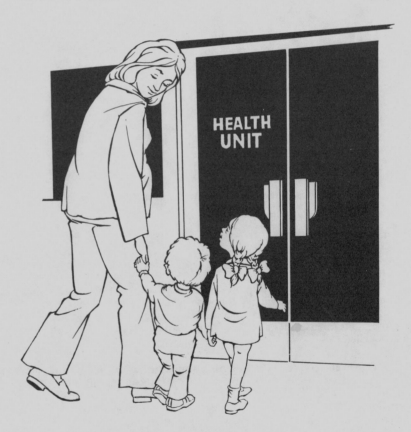

are well known and for this reason children receive vaccine against this disease early in life. Young women should be sure they have been vaccinated *before* becoming pregnant. However, if an expectant mother is unsure about having received the vaccine, the doctor can have a blood test done that tells whether sufficient protection is present. It is wise for expectant mothers to ensure that their preschool children have been vaccinated against rubella and encourage their friends to do likewise.

Unprotected expectant mothers should report any exposure to rubella to their physician.

## Coping with Stress:

Stress is a physical and emotional state that is always present in everybody and intensifies when changes or threats occur that require a response. Stress is increased during such times as sickness, loss of employment, marriage, change in residence and starting school. Pregnancy, with its physical changes, mood swings, financial adjustments and various other problems is a time of increased stress due to the emotional adjustments and lifestyle changes that must occur. Sometimes couples are unprepared to cope with these strains, especially if they have not foreseen the necessary changes in their pattern of living.

Since too much stress can become distress, ways of handling pressure have to be found. Some ways that can help:

- Talking with supportive friends, relatives, physician or nurse;

- Understanding what is happening and why these stressful feelings are occurring;

- Finding the best way to release frustration; for example, participating in a sport, reading a book, talking, or taking a walk;

- Planning ahead to avoid preventable crises or being prepared to cope with an unavoidable crisis;

- Learning to relax through such means as the relaxation exercises taught in prenatal classes and the various types of meditation.

It is important not to let stress build up, and so parents need to communicate with each other and to be able to talk together about their needs, frustrations and feelings.

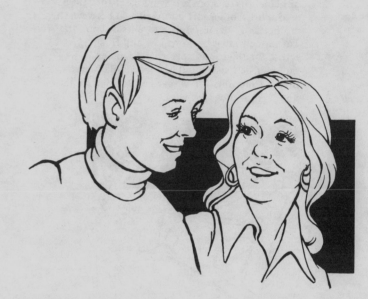

## Travel:

The decision about whether or not to travel depends upon the arduousness of the journey and the way the expectant mother feels. It is unwise to travel if ill, fatigued, or subject to dizzy spells.

Driving a car can continue as long as it is comfortable to sit behind the wheel. A short trip can be relaxing and a means of recreation, but long trips require planning so that the journey is safe and comfortable.

The following points should be considered when planning a trip:

- It is wise to consult the physician about travel especially in the first three and last months of pregnancy;

- Seat belts should be used when travelling by car or plane. Extensions are available if the seat belt is too short and a soft pillow placed between the mother and buckles/strap prevents discomfort. The lapbelt must be worn low and fit snugly across the thighs, not over the abdomen. The shoulder belt also should be worn in a car. British Columbia's new seat belt legislation does not exempt pregnant women;

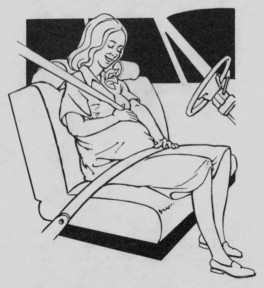

- On long trips, a rest stop every 160 kilometres (100 miles) or so helps to avoid fatigue. At that time it is also beneficial to take a short walk and to flex and contract the leg muscles;

- Some mothers find train or air travel less tiring than automobile travel. Each airline has their own regulations. At present, Air Canada requires a certificate from the doctor for travel in the ninth month. They will not accept expectant mothers within five days of the expected day of birth. Canadian Pacific Airlines require a special form to be completed by the physician if any complications exist and will not accept passengers after their eighth month of pregnancy. In any event, the airlines or travel agent should be consulted regarding their policies to avoid any problems with travel arrangements. It is sometimes difficult to land the plane at a good hospital ahead of the stork! If an expectant mother is travelling outside of North America, she should ensure that her polio immunizations are up-to-date. The need for any other vaccines should be discussed with the physician or health unit personnel. Under no circumstances should rubella or smallpox vaccine be given to a pregnant woman.

## Clothes:

"When I'm looking good, I'm feeling great" may be applicable to some women who find that dressing attractively contributes to their own and their family's good spirits. Other mothers feel that comfort is the main and only concern. Perhaps a compromise would be to select clothing for both comfort and appearance.

Clothes need not always be purchased new as a variety of clothes can be obtained by sewing, shopping at next-to-new shops and/or by exchanging items of clothing with friends. Something different to wear can be a real morale booster in the last month of pregnancy when waiting for delivery seems to be dragging. Many items can be worn after delivery if chosen with care. Maternity tops and front-opening sleepwear are especially useful for the breast-feeding mother.

The following suggestions may be helpful in selecting wearing apparel:

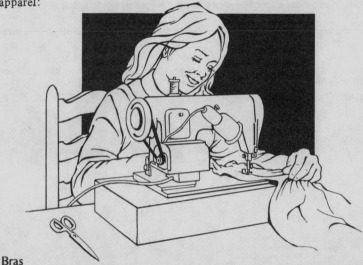

## Bras

During pregnancy, the gradually increasing size of the breasts necessitates buying progressively larger brassieres. A bra made of light weight material with wide straps will offer the best support and comfort and may also be worn at night.

In late pregnancy, nursing bras are a good buy as they can be used for breast-feeding later. Nursing bras come with both back and front openings, the choice of which is a matter of personal preference. A back closing bra is sometimes preferred as it affords support for one breast while nursing from the other. The nursing bra should be tried on before purchasing to check for comfort and ease in opening the flap with one hand (mother will want to be able to do this when holding the baby).

## Girdles

Women who are unaccustomed to wearing a girdle will probably not require one during pregnancy.

If a maternity girdle is necessary to provide support for the relief of backache as pregnancy advances, it should be of lightweight material, properly fitted, and not too tight. The legs should be loose and cutting "V's" in the sides will sometimes help.

## Hose

Maternity panty hose and specially designed garter belts are available, but elastic garters or knee-high hose are not advised as they can interfere with blood circulation and aggravate varicose veins. The doctor may prescribe support hose for varicose veins.

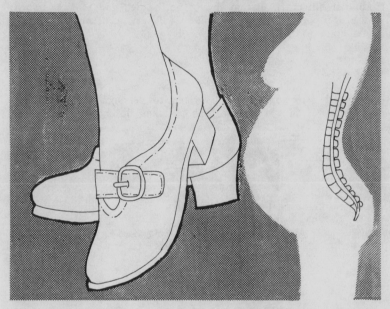

## Shoes

For comfort, a shoe that can support the extra weight is best. Shoes can be checked for support by placing the (empty) shoe on floor, and pressing down with thumb on the inner sole or shank (the part that comes under the arch). If the shoe gives under pressure, it will give weak support to the foot. Generally, a shoe with a broad, stable, low heel that provides good support can be worn for work. A 2" heel can be worn for dress if desired, but high heels tend to contribute to backache. On the other hand, a shoe that is too low such as a slipper or moccassin provides no support and may contribute to fatigue and aching legs and back. Bare feet in the sand, or for short periods indoors, can give relief to sore feet. Changing shoes during the day may also help.

### In Summary

Selecting a wardrobe from the wide variety of maternity and currently popular loose-fitting clothes can be fun. Loose, comfortable, non-constricting clothes that hang from the shoulder are most practical. Hose that hinder circulation should be avoided and footwear worn that gives support. Dress requirements will vary according to environmental conditions.

### Hygiene:

Special attention should be given to personal hygiene during pregnancy. A shower or bath can be taken throughout pregnancy,

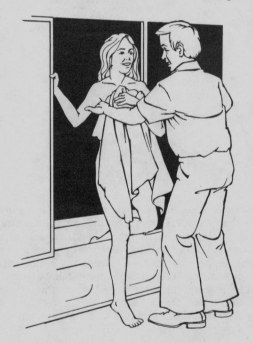

but in the last trimester, when the uterus becomes heavy, care must be taken against falling when getting in and out of bathtub.

During pregnancy the glands in the skin in the genital area are quite active and may give off an odor that some women find unpleasant. Washing with plain soap and water will keep the odor under control. Feminine deodorant sprays have been found to be irritating and so should be avoided. Douches should not be taken unless advised by the doctor.

**NOTES**

# CHAPTER 4
## DECISIONS

### Breast or Bottle?

To breast or bottle-feed is a decision every woman must make for herself. And although, for most, "breast is best", it is important that each mother wants to and knows why she has chosen to breast-feed. Or, if she makes the choice of bottle-feeding, the same thoughtfulness and understanding should have been involved.

### Reasons for breast-feeding
1. Breast milk is a real convenience food, readily available and germ free.

2. Breast milk is the right temperature day or night.

3. The fat, protein and salt content of breast milk makes it easier to digest than cow's milk or prepared formula.

4. Babies who are breast-fed are less susceptible to digestive upsets, infections, allergies.

5. Physically, the action of the sucking at the breasts leads to good development of teeth, jaw and palate.

6. Nursing speeds the return of the mother's uterus to its pre-pregnant state.

7. Emotionally, the intimate contact between the nursing infant and the mother helps to build a secure and loving relationship.

### Reasons for bottle-feeding
1. Some women may dislike the whole idea of a baby feeding from the breast.

2. Mothers who have already failed to breast-feed their first child may think it is not worth trying again.

3. A mother who has several children may think she just doesn't have time to breast-feed.

4. For others, it may be important to return to their work and thus it is difficult to fit breast-feeding into their daily schedule.

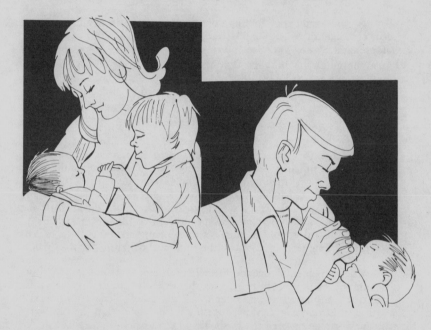

*In addition to the above facts*, the expectant mother is also influenced by the advice and opinions of others, her own experience in feeding previous babies but very especially, her partner's feelings.

Generally speaking, most women who wish to breast-feed are able to, providing they are helped to find ways around problems such as returning to work and coping with preschoolers. For example, the mother going out to work can breast-feed her baby in the morning and evening, leaving bottles of either formula or expressed breast milk, for the babysitter to give to the baby. When a busy toddler is about, the mother may like to put her free arm around him and visit or read a story while baby nurses. At other times, she may plan for the big brother or sister to play outside or to be sleeping while mother breast-feeds baby.

Further information on the management of breast-feeding is included in "Feeding and Care of the Baby", pages 76 to 79.

The importance of finding out answers to questions and exploring concerns cannot be overemphasized. Parents will have this opportunity at prenatal classes and also in visits to the physician and hospital. In many communities interested groups offer additional classes on breast-feeding and not to be overlooked is the selection of books available in libraries and bookstores, some of which are recommended at the end of this book.

### Changes in breasts during pregnancy

Tingling or tenderness of the breasts, due to hormonal activity, is one of the first signs of pregnancy. Breasts increase in size during pregnancy in preparation for producing milk to feed the infant. The areola, the area surrounding the nipple, enlarges and darkens and Montgomery's Tubercles become noticeable. These tubercles, or small glands (see Figure 1) secrete a thin lubricant which keeps the nipples soft, and blue veins become noticeable on the breast due to the extra blood supply required for the important task the breasts perform. Figure 1 illustrates the internal structure of the breast.

Until pregnancy occurs these structures are solid and without openings. As pregnancy progresses the alveoli (milk producing glands) and ducts are enlarging and opening. (The alveoli become hollow sacs with special openings that produce the milk. The milk is then collected in the ducts and stored in the sinuses until nursing occurs.) The baby's sucking stimulates what is known as the "let down reflex" which releases the milk and more milk is produced. During the last two or three months before the baby is born, the breasts may secrete a yellowish fluid called colostrum, the forerunner of milk. It is colostrum which the baby sucks for the first 2-3 days until the milk comes in.

### Care of the breasts during pregnancy

As the breasts enlarge, it is necessary to buy larger sized brassieres. A brassiere with wide shoulder straps provides comfort and support,

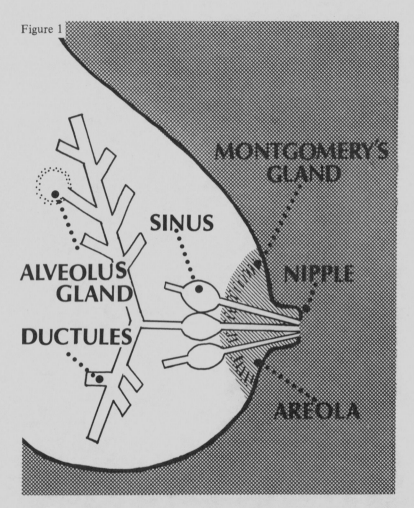

Figure 1

MONTGOMERY'S GLAND

SINUS

ALVEOLUS GLAND

NIPPLE

DUCTULES

AREOLA

and helps to prevent too much stretching of the tissues. Purchasing a nursing bra can be economical.

The breasts should be kept clean by washing with plain, warm water during the daily bath or shower. Soaps, especially perfumed ones, should be avoided as they remove the natural lubrication and can lead to irritated nipples.

## Preparation of the breasts for nursing

Even if the expectant mother can't decide how to feed her baby she can give her breasts special attention which will probably make breast-feeding easier and more enjoyable should she decide to give "nursing" a try. This involves:

### Strengthening and softening the nipples

The breasts can be prepared for nursing by several means and opinions vary about the methods. Generally, preparation to strengthen and keep the nipples soft can begin in the eighth month, but if the nipples seem flat or turned-in, the doctor should be consulted about the means to correct this early in the pregnancy. Strengthening the nipples may be accomplished by rubbing the breasts briskly but gently with a washcloth or towel after the bath and leaving the breasts uncovered for a few minutes each day.

Figure 2

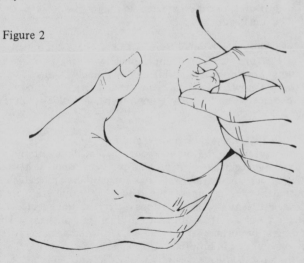

Several types of mild creams or oils, e.g., lanolin, baby oil, cold cream, or cocoa butter can be applied to the sides of the nipples

and areoli (but not over the duct openings) to make them soft. The cream or oil is placed on the fingers, the nipple pulled out gently and rolled between the thumb and forefinger, and the cream massaged gently around the nipple. By extending the nipple in this way, flat or slightly inverted nipples can be drawn out. Sometimes a nipple shield is recommended by the doctor. These are small plastic cups that can be worn under the brassiere and when worn daily for as many hours as possible should draw the nipple out. Usually shields can be obtained from the La Leché League or from a drugstore.

## Expressing Colostrum

The colostrum is an ideal first food for baby as it is thought to contain antibodies that give the breast-fed baby a resistance to disease.

Physicians are divided in their advice about prenatal expression of colostrum. Some recommend expressing a few drops daily, which will not deplete the supply, while others feel all colostrum should be saved for the first few feedings after birth.

Expressing colostrum in the last six to eight weeks of pregnancy should help the milk flow freely after the baby is born and prevent engorgement (back-up of milk causes breasts to become hard and hot).

Figure 3

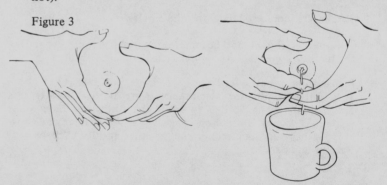

The technique for expressing colostrum is also handy to know since after baby is born the mother may wish to express milk into a bottle when she is going out without the baby or if engorgement does occur.

Colostrum is expressed in the following way:

- wash hands first;
- hold cup or cotton under the breast (or do in the shower);
- hold breast at the edge of the areola with thumb above and fingers beneath;
- push thumb and fingers together behind the nipple but do not slide fingers over the nipple;
- rotate hand back and forth a few times so that you reach all the milk ducts.

After expressing colostrum, dry the nipple and massage with a little cream or oil. A soft pad may be placed in the bra to catch any fluid oozing out of the breast. A plastic covering should never be used.

### Hints
Sometimes it is necessary to massage the breast to bring the colostrum or milk down. This is done by placing the fingers flatly on the breast near the chest wall and sliding the fingers along the ducts. This brings the colostrum or milk from the alveoli along the ducts to the reservoir. See Figure 3.

The fingers should *not* slide over the nipples.

The mother should not become discouraged if nothing happens the first few times this procedure is tried as practice helps.

### Preparation for bottle-feeding
Just as it is helpful for all mothers to prepare their breasts, it is also helpful for all mothers to know about bottle-feeding. What equipment to buy is listed on page 41 of this chapter while how to feed baby is discussed in the chapter entitled, "Baby Feeding and Care".

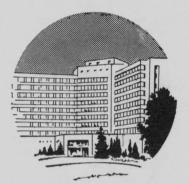

## Hospital or Home?

In recent years home deliveries have captured the imagination of the mass media as a new development in maternity care. Ironically, the trend is not really new but the resurgence of a custom that was once a necessity. Before hospital and medical insurance became available, many Canadians could not afford to go to a hospital. In addition, hospitals were not always accessible. Today the availability and accessibility of medical and hospital care are no longer problems except in very isolated circumstances.

In many hospitals, personnel have rallied to rectify the accusation that their care is too sterile and impersonal by trying to make their maternity units more homelike and family centered. Changes in policy in some hospitals now allow fathers in the delivery room, parents to have more contact with the baby (rooming-in), and older children to visit mother in hospital.

Over the years, advances in medical and nursing knowledge and the availability of equipment and other resources coinciding with the trend for births to take place in the protected hospital environment have had a very positive effect on the survival rates for mothers and babies. Although most deliveries are uneventful, today's hospital staff are prepared to deal efficiently with situations that arise unexpectedly and which could present a critical threat to mother and/or baby. This is perhaps the most important aspect to consider, when deciding whether to give birth at home or in hospital. Although the decision about where to give birth must be made with the doctor who will attend the delivery, it is the parents who must ultimately make the decision and then share the responsibility for the outcome of their decision.

## What to Get Ready for the Baby:

The furniture, clothing and equipment that must be prepared in advance for the baby will depend upon space available, personal preferences, finances, and community customs. The most important consideration in selecting the items should be safety and comfort.

To new parents, the list included here may seem long but the baby's wardrobe and equipment need not be new. Many items might be obtained from friends, relatives, next-to-new shops, sales, or home-made. Gifts are frequently received for the first baby, and so it is wise to prepare only the necessities in advance of delivery. The following information is included to provide guidance in obtaining articles needed for the baby.

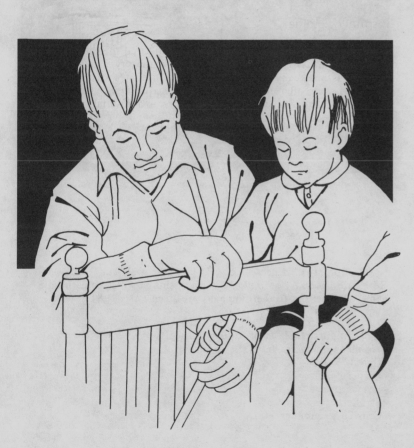

### Furniture
- Crib, bassinet, laundry basket, sturdy box or carriage to sleep in.
- Infant car seat for travel (see page 43).
- Diaper pail with a lid.
- Drawers or box to store clothing in.
- A rocking chair, although not essential, is certainly pleasurable for both mother and baby.

### Clothing
The clothing required will vary according to climate and laundry facilities. As the baby grows quickly, it is advisable to purchase infant sizes six months to one year.

*Diapers* – 3 to 4 dozen. If using a diaper service only one dozen is needed for emergencies. No more than one package of disposable diapers should be purchased in case baby is unable to wear them.

*Undershirts* – 4. Avoid buttons down the front or tight neckbands. Front ties or grippers are easiest to put on or shirts with extra shoulder opening space. AVOID BUTTONS.

*Nightgowns* – 3 or 4 or sleepers.

*Receiving Blankets* – 3 or 4. Useful for crib blankets and wrapping baby while feeding.

*Quilted Crib Pads* – 4. Make sure that one side is waterproof.

*Mattress Protector* – 1. See section 44.

*Crib Sheets* – 4. Fitted are easiest. Ordinary sheets can be converted by mitering corners and sewing. Pillow cases may be used for bassinet or carriage.

*Sweater* – 1.

*Baby Blankets* – 2. (depending on the season)

*Waterproof Pants* – 3 or 4.

*Bibs* – 2 or 3.

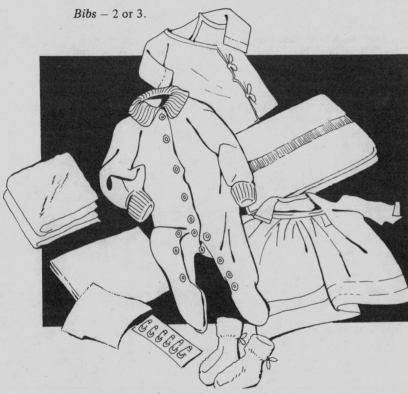

### Bath Equipment
A box or tray may be prepared for the baby's bath. It can contain:

- Mild soap in a dish;
- Cotton balls in a jar (avoid cotton tipped applicators as a sharp poke can hurt delicate tissues);

- Alcohol for cleaning around the cord, if recommended ;
- Diaper pins with safety metal ends (so they don't open unexpectedly);
- *Optional* - vaseline or non-perfumed oil for buttocks.
  - powder (cornstarch or unscented talcum).

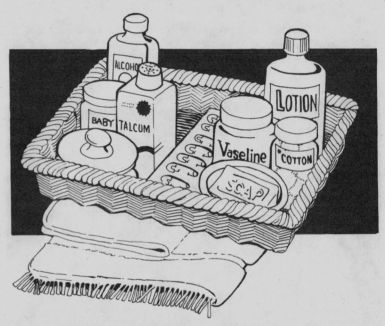

In addition, two large soft towels or bathtowels and two washcloths are necessary as well as a basin or sink in which to bathe the baby. Instructions for bathing baby are given on page 81.

### Things to purchase later or to suggest as gifts
- Woollens - sweaters, bonnets, booties
- Cuddle Seat
- Diaper Bag
- Baby Carriage
- Stroller
- Crib Toys - mobiles, etc.

- Baby spoon, dish, and cup
- Back-pack or carrying pouch for baby.

## Feeding Equipment

The supplies required will depend upon whether the baby is breast-fed or bottle-fed, and the appliances available in the home, such as refrigerator and dishwasher. The formula should be sterilized until the baby is six weeks old, or for longer if the purity of the water supply is questionable.

Disposable equipment and kits with bottles and sterilizing pots are available to the consumer. Only one or two bottles will be needed if breast-feeding. Generally, the following list meets the need for bottle-feeding.

- 6 to 8 large bottles and nipples
- 1 or 2 small bottles

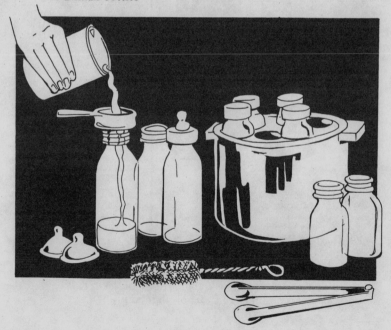

- Bottle brush
- Funnel
- Tongs
- Sterilizer pot or large canning pot — not necessary if dishwasher is available.

Instructions on preparation of the formula can be found on page 80.

## Toys

Sometimes the first item purchased for the new baby is a toy as an expression of the parents' joy in anticipation of the baby's arrival. Because toys serve a useful purpose, parents should be knowledgeable about the types to purchase as well as the safety of the toys.

As babies learn by actively experimenting on the world around them, it is important that they have the stimulation of suitable materials in their environment even before they can move about to explore for themselves. Early learning is done through the senses — seeing, hearing, touching, and tasting. Knowing this, parents are in a position to choose toys which provide some of the stimulation their baby needs to learn and grow.

Some examples of toys suitable for the new baby from birth to six months are: rattles, large plastic rings, crib mobiles, hanging unbreakable mirrors, bells, music boxes with moving figures, rattling or squeaking toys, small soft animals, plastic or rubber blocks with rounded edges, and strings of coloured spools or large plastic beads.

Toys should be selected for safety as well as play value. The better manufacturers test their toys and provide a written statement of their product's safety.

A safe toy should be:
- Sturdy;
- Washable;
- Without sharp or rough edges even when broken;
- Non-inflammable;
- Small enough to be held easily and manipulated;
- Large enough not to go in the baby's mouth,
- Have no detachable parts that can be swallowed or cause other injuries;

- Painted or dyed with non-toxic materials.

Additional hints on toy buying may be obtained by writing to:

Canadian Toy Testing Council
Box 6014, Station J
Ottawa, Ontario
K2A 1T1

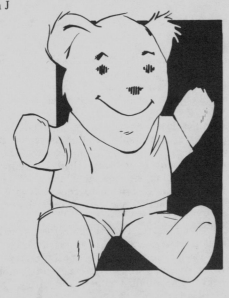

## Pacifiers

During the first two months of life the newborn infant has a great need to suck and usually will suck on anything that comes in contact with the lips. If a pacifier is used, it should:

- be made of a material that will withstand boiling;
- have a shield large and rigid enough to prevent the nipple from going too far into the baby's mouth;
- be made in one piece to avoid nipple coming off shield;
- be made of non-toxic material and empty of water or fluid that might be contaminated;
- be sterile at the time of purchase;
- have cord no longer than 4" – 6" (long cords from soothers can strangle the baby).

The following diagrams can be used to test pacifiers or rattles to ensure that their measurements are safe.

### How to Test for Safety of Pacifier or Rattles

1. Draw Diagram A according to given measurements and paste on cardboard.
2. Cut out gauge opening.
3. Fold at dotted lines.
4. Set gauge on flat surface.
5. Insert rattle as illustrated in Diagram B.

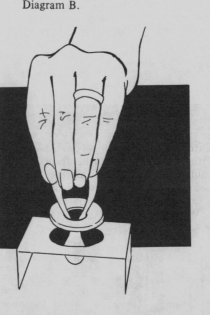

1 3/16"  30 mm

FOLD LINE

35mm. (1 3/8")

CUT OUT

50 mm. (1 15/16")

FOLD LINE

▲ Diagram B          Diagram A ▶

6. If rattle or component passes through gauge and touches the edge of the opening – the rattle is too small to be safe and is unsuitable for use by an infant.

42

The seat has a safety harness for the baby and is held secure by the car's lap belt. The Consumer Reports magazine and the Department of Consumer and Corporate Affairs have up-to-date information on suitable models to purchase according to the child's weight and age.

Car seats, approved by the Consumer Association of Canada, are the best buy. The label should state: "This product complies with applicable requirements of the Children's Car Seats and Harnesses Regulations". To be approved a seat must meet three basic criteria.

(a) It must restrain the child.

(b) There must be no breakage on collision that might injure the child.

(c) The seat must not twist so as to trap the child.

Car seats vary in price and effectiveness and unless all the manufacturer's instructions are followed, the device becomes virtually useless. Pictures of appropriate car seats are included below.

## Car Seats

For parents who use an automobile or truck for transporation, the provision of a car seat for the baby should be decided upon before birth as infants should ride in an infant car seat, even on their first trip from the hospital. Infants and small children are so vulnerable that even a minor accident, which would only bruise an adult, can kill a child. The baby is not safe in the mother's arms as the child can be wrenched from her arms by the force of impact in an accident. Car beds and household infant seats are not designed to protect in a crash.

The infant will be safe and comfortable in the semi-reclining position of a car carrier which will not harm the infant's back. Newborns seem more comfortable with rolled blankets to pad the carrier sides.

A rearward-facing device as shown at right is preferable for infants.

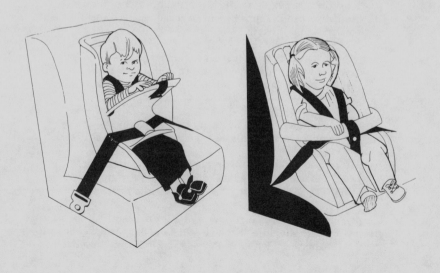

## Cribs and Cradles

When deciding what to put the baby to sleep in — crib, cradle, drawer, carriage, or playpen, it is well to keep in mind that legislation was enacted in 1974 to make cribs and cradles safer. These standards were designed to prevent serious accidents which sometimes happened with older models. Parents can make an older crib safe with a few simple adjustments. Easy instructions on how to do this can be obtained by mailing the attached coupon to: B.C. Ministry of Health, Division of Health Promotion & Information, Victoria.

The following are some sensible safety rules to consider when preparing the baby's sleeping accommodation.

(a) The place selected should be away from drafts, cold walls, radiators or hot air ducts.

(b) The vertical bars on the crib should be so close to one another that even the smallest head will not fit through them.

(c) The mattress must be firm (a hard pillow or a folded pad made from quilt or blanket could be used for a mattress). It should fit closely to sides, top and bottom of the crib so baby's head cannot become wedged between the mattress and the crib.

(d) The mattress can be set at a position comfortable for the mother when the baby is newborn, but near the floor when there is danger of the baby rolling over or climbing out.

(e) Loose pillows are not necessary and should be avoided as lying on a flat surface is best for the baby's bone structure.

(f) It is a good idea to develop the habit of keeping large toys and articles out of the crib. As the baby grows they can be used as steps to climb over the sides.

Usually the type of bassinet or crib that is used at first is soon outgrown. Parents should realize that when the baby is tall enough to stand with the shoulders over the side rail it is time to move to a larger crib.

Date . . . . . . . . . . . . . . . . .

Please send me directions for making an older crib safe.

Name . . . . . . . . . . . . . . . . . . . . . . . . . . . . . . . .
(Please print clearly)

Address . . . . . . . . . . . . . . . . . . . . . . . . . . . . . . . .

. . . . . . . . . . . . . . . . . . . . . . . Postal Code . . . . . . . . . . .

Mail to:      B.C. Ministry of Health
              Division of Health Promotion & Information
              1515 Blanshard Street
              Victoria, B.C.
              V8W 3C8

## Playpens

Playpens are used sometimes as a substitute for a crib. Parents should be aware of the regulations for design, construction, and performance of playpens, under the Hazardous Products Act that became effective September 1, 1976. It is now illegal to sell a playpen, new or used, which does not meet these specifications.

(a) The mesh must be small and strong enough to prevent a child from getting a finger ensnarled in it. Mosquito netting size is acceptable.

(b) No playpen should have more than two wheels or coasters to prevent the playpen from rolling away.

(c) All playpens must pass government stability tests.

(d) All metal parts must be free from rough and sharp edges.

(e) Exposed wooden or plastic parts must be smoothly finished.

Older wooden playpens can be made safe by following the same instructions as for cribs. The rules for sensible crib safety are also applicable.

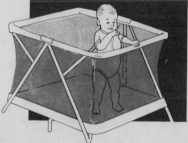

## How to Prepare the Other Children:

Even if the child is too young to understand the changes which a brother or sister will bring, the parents should talk about the baby's arrival. To any child, the months seem long, and so, most parents wait until the fourth or fifth month to ask, "Have you noticed mummy's tummy getting bigger?" Reactions to this news will vary and parents should not be surprised if their child is less than enthusiastic about the future baby. After all, a brother or sister means giving up some of mother's and father's love as well as the attention of "important others" such as granny and grandpa.

Expecting a baby provides parents with a natural way of talking with older preschoolers about "where babies come from". A question such as, "Do you remember when Mrs. Smith had a big tummy and there was a baby inside? Well, mummy's going to have a baby too." can be a good starting point.

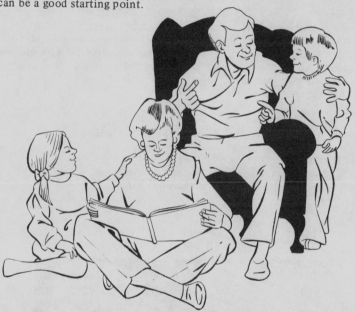

Looking at books* together and providing opportunity through play, are two ways parents can help their children to talk and to express their feelings about the baby. It is also helpful and fun to involve all the family in fixing up baby's furniture and clothes.

Any changes which could be interpreted as rejection or discrimination, if they coincided with baby's arrival, should be made well in advance. For example, if a child is of nursery-school age, it is wise

*See Suggested Reading page 107.

to send him well before baby's arrival, so that he meets other people and doesn't feel "pushed-out", as he might, if starting school coincided with baby's birth. Moving from a crib to a bed or giving up certain clothes, toys or other equipment are examples of other changes which may have to be made well ahead of Birth Day. Many mothers like to have tucked in their suitcase, a little gift from the baby for the brother or sister who comes to visit in the hospital, or on arrival home.

But most important, both before and after baby's arrival, is planning a special time that belongs to each child. And since there are so many demands on the expectant and new mother's time, she must plan her day ahead to do this. While some mothers choose a walk or some physical activity to enjoy together, others find that a quiet time spent reading, visiting, and even falling asleep pleases the child and provides mother with needed rest.

## What to Get Ready Before Going to the Hospital:

### The Household

Plans will have to be made for organizing the household before mother goes to the hospital. If there are other children in the family,

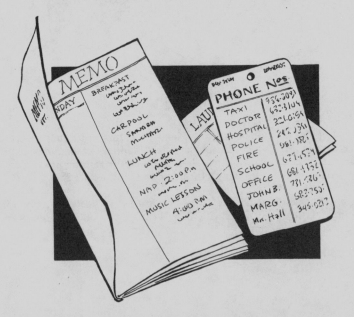

arrangements for their care will be dependent upon their ages, schooling and help available. Preparations cannot be left until the last minute even if, father, a homemaker service, or grandparents are being depended upon.

Detailed written instructions about the children's care should be prepared. The instructions should include the daily routine of meals, naps, bedtime, school, music lessons, car pools, emergency telephone numbers, and other relevant information. Food preferences and practices regarding such items as "junk foods", safety, and any "not allowed" activities should be included as well.

By the eighth month of pregnancy emergency telephone numbers should be prominently displayed by the telephone and should remain for the babysitter's use. The list should include the following numbers:

Taxi
Family doctor and any specialists giving care
Hospital
Fire
Police
Ambulance
Poison Control
Father's place of business
Nearest friend or relative

It is important to arrange who will drive the mother to hospital and to have an alternate driver available.

If the family car is to be used for the trip to the hospital, it should have ample gas in the tank and be ready to go both day and night.

The room or space that is set aside for the baby will need to be prepared in advance. The clothing, equipment and furniture need to be purchased or borrowed and made ready for use. The baby's clothes need to be laundered to remove excess lint and ensure softness (before being put into drawers). Mild soap flakes or a mild biodegradable detergent are best. Laundry products such as strong detergents, bleach and softeners may irritate the baby's skin. In any case, thorough rinsing of the laundry is important to avoid skin irritation.

## Items to be packed and left at home

Going home clothes can be left ready for father to bring to hospital as storage space usually is very limited.

**For baby:** Shirt and gown or sleepers
Diapers and pins
Plastic pants
Sweater, bonnet and booties (if wearing a gown)
Shawl or blanket — bunting bag depending upon weather

**For mother:** Loose fitting clothes, comfortable and convenient for breast-feeding.

Many mothers wear maternity clothes home as former clothes may be rather snug since not all weight gained is lost immediately.

## Items to take to hospital

The following list varies according to individual preferences, hospital and method of childbirth used. The items suggested here can be used as a guide although not all may be necessary.

**Grooming aides:** Additional to normal cosmetics

deodorant                     nail file
soap*                         lotion for skin*
dusting powder                mouth freshener*
toothbrush and paste          shower cap
dental floss                  shampoo

## Clothing

slippers with backs that       panties
  give support                 pyjama bottoms or slacks for
a bed jacket or sweater **       postnatal exercises
a washable dressing gown       socks
a nightgown* or pyjamas **     sanitary belt and pads*
maternity bras (2 or 3)

## Extras

facial tissues*
soap for washing bra
stationery (pen, stamps, address book)
announcement cards can be bought at most hospitals

## Labor Kit

articles suggested by prenatal instructor can be listed here

\* articles supplied by some hospitals.
\*\* front opening if breast-feeding is planned.

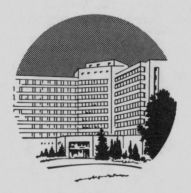

- The pubic hair is usually shaved or clipped to cleanse the area, but this practice is changing and not all doctors consider it to be necessary now.

- An enema is usually given unless the patient has had diarrhea or a bowel movement prior to admission.

- An intravenous infusion is started routinely in some hospitals on all patients in labor; in others this is not done.

- Artificial rupture of the membranes (amniotomy) is done by some doctors and parents will want to know when and how this is done.

## Questions to Ask the Doctor or Hospital Staff:

1. **Are hospital tours available?**
   Information about the hospital is generally included in prenatal classes and a tour of the maternity unit is frequently provided.

   The supervisor or head nurse of the maternity unit will sometimes arrange for tours for parents who are not attending classes. The policy regarding tours can be ascertained locally by telephoning the hospital or health unit.

2. **Is pre-registration necessary?**
   Many hospitals prefer expectant parents to register at a convenient time in advance. This provides information for the hospital and avoids delay for the parents during admission after labor has begun. Particulars regarding Medical and Hospital Coverage will be needed when pre-registering at the hospital.

3. **What are the routine admission procedures?**
   Sometimes couples become separated temporarily, during the hospital admission procedures and if this is a possibility the staff should be told that the parents wish to be reunited.

   Further information about the following routines can be obtained:

   - Blood and urine specimens are generally collected on admission, but if labor is too far advanced, this may be done after delivery.

4. **Is father allowed in the labor and delivery rooms?**
   The father who wishes to be present in the delivery room will need to discuss this with the physician early in pregnancy. The father will need to make arrangements to leave work on short notice as well.

5. **Is there flexibility in the positions that can be used during delivery?**
   Some women find pushing difficult while lying in the lithotomy position as shown in Figure 4, with the feet in stirrups. A back rest or the addition of two pillows under the back may be more comfortable. The positions can be tried in prenatal classes and the mother's preference discussed with the physician.

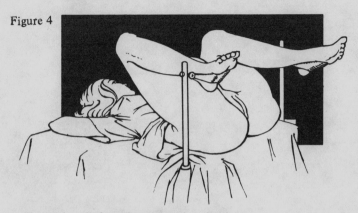

Figure 4

### 6. What pain relief medications are available?

The doctor can also be asked about the availability of pain relief medication, the types of anaesthetic used during the delivery process, and the reactions that may be expected. Preferences can be made known to the doctor, realizing though, that the doctor may have to make alternate decisions during labor about the type of pain relief medication or anaesthetic to be used. The mother who may not wish to have any medication should remember that it is available to her if she changes her mind or is having difficulty coping on her own.

### 7. Is an episiotomy necessary?

An episiotomy is an incision made at the opening of the vagina to facilitate the birth of the baby's head and avoid tearing of the perineal area. Recently, some books and magazine articles have appeared about the use and misuse of this procedure. The opponents claim that the procedure is done too frequently and that it is not always necessary. Some mothers have felt they experienced unnecessary discomfort associated with the healing of the incision. The pain adversely affected their marital relationships as intercourse was feared and was painful for some time afterwards.

Many physicians feel an episiotomy should be done to avoid tearing which is more difficult to repair than a clean incision. The other reasons for doing an episiotomy is to prevent damage to the baby's head and also to avoid weakness in the mother's perineal area in later life.

A local anaesthetic is used for this procedure and the sutures are of a material that dissolves so removal is not necessary. Special care is usually given to the incision while mother is in hospital.

The expectant parents should discuss the issue with their physician so that an understanding can be reached.

### 8. Is rooming-in available?

Rooming-in is an arrangement, available in many maternity units, whereby the mother and baby share accommodations and the mother cares for the baby under the guidance of the nurse. Rooming-in may be modified to have baby in the nursery at regular intervals (for example, at night), or upon request of the mother. The baby is also physically accessible to the father to hold, caress and enjoy. The mother can learn a great deal about the baby's sleep-wake patterns and physical needs. The baby begins to learn about his parents and how they respond to his needs. This close family togetherness also enables the mother and father to discover how they feel about each other. It is, in fact, the birth of a family.

Although the mother rooms-in with the baby, she is not totally responsible for the care twenty-four hours of the day. The hospital staff are available to provide relief and act as consultants and teachers, so the mother gains confidence and competence in caring for the baby.

The decision about whether to use this type of hospital accommodation should be the parents' choice unless medical complications require other arrangements.

### 9. What is the best way to begin parent-infant bonding?

Bonding, or attachment, is defined as "a unique relationship between two people that is specific and endures through time". Although it isn't known how attachment bonds are actually formed, it is helpful to realize that many factors combine to influence the parent-infant bonding process. They include the parents' genetic, cultural and socioeconomic background, personalities, present and past pregnancy experiences and the circumstances of the present labor and delivery such as length of labor, medical crisis during labor, obstetrical medication and baby's health and condition at birth.

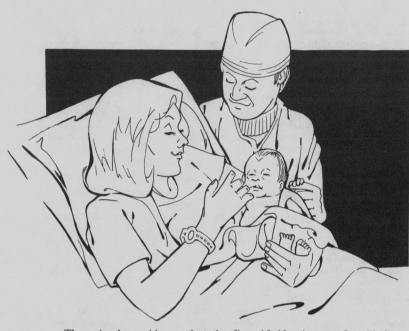

There is also evidence that the first 45-60 minutes after birth are an especially sensitive period when the bonding process can be enhanced. At this time the baby is in a "quiet alert" state and responds to his parents' caressing, talking and eye-to-eye contact with him. However, it is also important to realize that close, loving maternal and paternal bonds with baby can be established later by parents who have to be separated from their newborn and by adoptive parents.

It is suggested that parents talk to their physician about their desire for early contact with their newborn. Questions on the topic can also be brought up at prenatal class and on the hospital tour.

CHAPTER 5

# SOME MEDICAL CONSIDERATIONS AND PROCEDURES IN PREGNANCY

The medical management of a pregnancy is dependent upon the individual doctor's method of practice. This chapter deals with medical considerations that sometimes occur in pregnancy.

## Blood Incompatibility:

Each person has blood of one of four groups: — O, A, B or AB. In addition, the blood may contain the Rhesus (Rh) antigen, and is called Rh positive (Rh+). Blood without the factor is called Rh negative (Rh-).

The two most common blood incompatibilities which may occur between mother and father are *Rh Incompatibility* (when the baby of an Rh- mother inherits the father's Rh+ blood) and *ABO Incompatibility* (when the baby inherits a different ABO group from that of the mother).

### Rh Incompatibility
This problem will occur only when the fetus inherits the Rh+ factor from the father (as shown in the following chart) and the Rh-mother develops antibodies to reject it.

## BLOOD FACTORS

|    | Mother | Father | Baby (Fetus) | Problem |
|----|--------|--------|--------------|---------|
| 1. | Rh- | Rh- | Rh- | No |
| 2. | Rh+ | Rh+ | Rh+ | No |
| 3. | Rh+ | Rh- | Rh+ or - | No |
| 4. | Rh- | Rh+ | Rh- | No |
| 5. | Rh- | Rh+ | Rh+ | Maybe |

This problem has been reduced in incidence to only once in 2500 births since the introduction of immune globulin, an Rh vaccine which is given to the Rh- mother by injection shortly after the first Rh+ baby is born or after each miscarriage or abortion. This injection prevents the mother from producing antibodies which may cause a problem in future pregnancies, but is unlikely to help if the mother has already become sensitized to the Rh antigen.

Fortunately, the physician can monitor the mother's blood and amniotic fluid prenatally and the baby's blood and clinical condition postnatally. Observation of the baby includes watching for jaundice or yellowing of the skin and the white part of the eyes. If treatment is required, one of the measures used is placement of the baby under a light of increased intensity with his eyes covered for protection. The purpose of this procedure is to make the bilirubin (substance causing the jaundice) less toxic and more easily excreted. An exchange blood transfusion is necessary when the amount of bilirubin continues to increase more quickly than it should.

### ABO Incompatibility
An incompatibility may arise when the baby's blood grouping is different from the mother's in relation to A, B, AB, and O types. This condition cannot be detected until after birth but the clinical effect is usually less severe than Rh incompatibility, and as a result, requires treatment in relatively fewer babies. If necessary, an exchange blood transfusion may have to be given.

## Amniocentesis:

Amniocentesis is performed by the physician to obtain a sample of amniotic fluid which is withdrawn into a syringe after passing a needle through the mother's abdomen into the uterus. This procedure is done only in special circumstances when the results are necessary to check on the health of the fetus or to detect inherited or other congenital problems. Amniocentesis may be undertaken in the fourth month of pregnancy. The test can be done later in pregnancy to monitor the well-being of a fetus whose mother and father have different Rh blood groups. Near term, the test can assist in determining the gestational age of the fetus and in ruling out an inadequate amount of surfactant necessary for baby's survival outside the mother's body. This information is important in complicated pregnancies where early delivery may be considered necessary.

## Caesarian Birth:

A caesarian birth is the delivery of the baby through an incision made into the mother's abdomen and uterus. The operation is called a caesarian section, the word coming from the Latin "caedere" meaning to cut. There is no proof to substantiate the claim that Julius Caesar was born by this means, but the records do show that a successful "C - section" took place in Switzerland in the year 1500.

The purpose of performing the section is to preserve the life or health of the mother and/or her fetus. The most common reason for the caesarian delivery is when the baby's head is too large to pass through the mother's birth canal. Such disproportion can be determined by x-ray, internal examinations, and by sonography, which shows the size and position of the fetus. From these and other test results, parents can know in advance if the baby is to be delivered by caesarian section, but other times, the need for surgical intervention may not be determined until labor begins.

Other reasons for caesarian births include failure of the labor to progress normally, certain changes of fetal heart rate pattern, medical factors involving the mother, and position of the baby, placenta or umbilical cord. If a mother has had a caesarian birth, further babies nearly always are delivered in the same way, but this depends upon the individual case and reason why the section was done.

The mother who wishes to remain alert during the operation should discuss this with the doctor because either spinal or general anaesthetics may be used.

Parents should also attend prenatal classes and let the instructor know that they will be having a caesarian birth so that the class can meet their learning needs. As over 13%* of all births in British Columbia are delivered by caesarian section, some health units have been providing classes on this topic. Some hospitals give preparation classes for these deliveries too.

The mother's stay in hospital may be two or three days longer with a caesarian delivery, but breast-feeding and rooming-in usually are not affected. To facilitate observation the baby may be kept in an incubator for a few hours, but brought to the mother for feeding.

## Sonography (Ultrasound):

Sonography is a diagnostic technique where high frequency sound waves, produced in a machine, are applied to the mother's abdomen. The waves pass through soft tissue such as the wall of the uterus, but are partially reflected by the placenta and fetus. The reflections form a two-dimensional picture. This picture helps the physician to determine the gestational age and to monitor the growth of the fetus. The position of the placenta can also be identified.

Sonography equipment is available in many hospitals. The procedure is simple, painless and free of risk to mother or fetus.

## Breech Delivery:

Breech is a term applied to the position of the fetus when a part (feet, arm, buttocks, hip) of the body other than the head settles down into the mother's pelvic cavity. As a result, the labor may be prolonged because the presenting part is soft and therefore does not help to dilate the cervix as efficiently as if the presenting part had been the head. Sometimes the doctor will try to turn the fetus or provide other obstetrical help, such as caesarian section, depending upon the individual circumstances.

3-4% of all deliveries are breech births and in one third of all twin births, at least one fetus will be in breech presentation (Reeder p. 498).

*Physicians' Notices of Birth, 1976. B.C. Ministry of Health.

## Twins:

Twins (the presence of two fetuses in the uterus) are the most commonly occurring form of multiple pregnancy. Twins are *identical* if both fetuses develop from one ovum which was fertilized by one sperm from the father. *Fraternal* twins occur when two ova have been fertilized by two sperm and therefore only resemble each other as members of the same family.

In about 75% of cases, presence of twins can be confirmed by sonography by the second month of pregnancy.

Two main considerations with multiple pregnancies are the position of the fetuses and the mother's ability to carry them to term. Frequently twins are born about two weeks early and tend to be of lower birth weight than single births.

The mother who is carrying twins may find her abdomen larger than with a single fetus, and as the pregnancy advances, experience more movement. For fullest fetal growth achievement, and to minimize the chance of premature onset of labor, the mother should have more rest and extra attention to diet.

The method selected for delivery will depend upon a number of factors such as the number of previous children the mother has had, the size of the mother's pelvis and the fetal positions and sizes.

## Stress Test (Oxytocin Challenge Test):

The stress test is used to obtain information about the fetal ability to tolerate labor. Carefully measured amounts of oxytocin are given using an intravenous infusion pump to the mother while the fetal monitor records the fetal heart beat pattern. This test is usually used when an induced labor is being considered.

## Electronic Monitoring (External and Internal):

Monitoring the frequency, intensity and duration of contractions and their effect on fetal heart rate patterns with electronic equipment gives an accurate picture of the health status of the fetus and the uterus during labor. Possible problems can be identified early before they become a threat to the mother or fetus.

Some doctors monitor all patients. Others use it during induction, or when the mother has medical problems such as diabetes, toxemia, or heart disease, or if she has had labor problems previously. Monitoring may be done either externally or internally.

### External
External electronic monitoring in done by gently strapping small, sensitive transducers on the mother's abdomen. The transmission of fetal heart sounds is recorded on a moving graph paper and can be interpreted as heart rate by the nurses and doctors.

Although the prevailing preference is for the mother to lie on her side, she can adjust her position for comfort and practice breathing for relaxation. She may be disconnected from the monitor to go to the bathroom or for a walk.

### Internal
Internal monitoring is used once actual labor has begun and the membranes have ruptured. Thin, soft plastic tubing is inserted through the cervix alongside the fetal head during a vaginal examination. The tube is attached to the monitor to accurately measure changes in pressure within the uterus during contractions.

In addition, a small electrode is attached to the fetal scalp and connected to the monitor with thin wires to transmit the electrocardiac activity of the fetus. The electrode will not harm the fetus. The small marks from the electrode will disappear in two or three days.

Although she must be on her side most of the time, the mother usually finds internal monitoring more comfortable because it is less cumbersome than having the belt over her tummy. The one restriction is that she will be confined to using a bedpan instead of going to the bathroom.

## Stethoscope and Fetoscope:

When electronic monitoring is not used, the nurse listens to the fetal heart rate with a stethoscope or fetoscope at regular intervals.

## Induction:

Induction is the stimulation of labor before it would begin spontaneously. In other words, sometimes nature needs a nudge and labor must be induced by the doctor. Very few women deliver on the date they are due as some may be two weeks early while others may be two weeks late; therefore, a mother shouldn't expect to be induced if the baby does not arrive on the expected date.

There are two common methods of induction. One is by intravenous infusion of carefully controlled amounts of oxytocin, a medication which causes the uterus to contract. The success of the procedure depends on many factors, including the maturity of the baby, the number of weeks of pregnancy, and the readiness of the patient's cervix to dilate. Inductions performed by intravenous infusion are termed "medical" inductions.

The second mode of induction is by rupturing the bag of fluid around the baby. This causes the uterus to contract and often initiates labor. This is perhaps the simplest method of induction. Once again, it must be carefully evaluated by the doctor if it is to be successful.

A physician may rupture the membranes and also use oxytocin which is very effective in inducing labor. Indications for induction vary but the main reason must be concern for what is best for the mother and child.

## Forceps:

Forceps are spoon-like instruments that sometimes are placed on either side of the fetal head to protect it, and sometimes to ease the delivery by using traction and rotation. Forceps were used for many centuries to assist complicated labors before caesarian sections became safer and easier for both mother and child. Nowadays, forceps are still used in certain situations.

Sometimes forceps leave red marks on the side of the baby's head. No treatment is required as the marks begin to fade within a few days of the baby's birth.

## Prematurity — Low Birth Weight:

Babies delivered before the 37th week of gestation are considered preterm. Infants with a birthweight of 2,500 grams or less are usually immature. Some low birthweight infants may be quite mature, even full-term, but small because of some growth problems during the pregnancy. Although babies weighing less than 1,000 grams can survive under highly specialized and constant care, the lower the birthweight the higher the mortality rate. It is the most premature babies that have the highest risk of developing respiratory distress syndrome. This is due to the immaturity of the lungs and the inability to keep the air spaces open.

In recent years, several forms of therapy have been used to avoid the problems of prematurity and immaturity. A number of tests on amniotic fluid obtained by amniocentesis will allow the physician to predict the immature baby's ability to breathe effectively if delivery is imminent. The physician may attempt to maintain the pregnancy by using a drug to delay the delivery of the premature baby until the lungs have matured. The closer the pregnancy comes to the full-term expected date of delivery the less the risk to the newborn.

## Regional Perinatal Resources:

Pregnancy and childbirth are natural, mainly happy processes, and should be treated as such. They should not be treated as a disease. Occasionally, a doctor or nurse can recognize circumstances that carry a predictable risk of complication, either for the mother or for the baby. It may be that the facilities for meeting the mother's or baby's special needs are not available in the local community hospital. Under these circumstances, it is safer for the delivery to take place in a referral hospital, where these resources are immediately at hand.

Certain hospitals in the province have been designated as regional referral centres where pregnant women with a predicted risk may be cared for in a setting which provides special expertise and resources for the mother and infant.

Even with the best predictions, some babies will be born with an unexpected complication requiring specialized facilities for newborn diagnosis or intensive care. If such a problem arises in a community hospital, a transport service for the baby is in operation to maintain good care of such an infant during the journey to the regional neonatal special care unit.

**NOTES**

**NOTES**

55

CHAPTER 6

## GIVING BIRTH

## Signs of Forthcoming Labor:

Lightening occurs two to three weeks before the onset of labor. The fetus slips down into the pelvis thereby relieving the pressure on the diaphragm and mother experiences increased frequency of urination from the increased pressure on the bladder.

By the end of the ninth month the fetal head usually has become engaged; that is, it is in a position ready for birth lying between the mother's pubic bone and the sacrum (lower part of spine) as shown in the picture below.

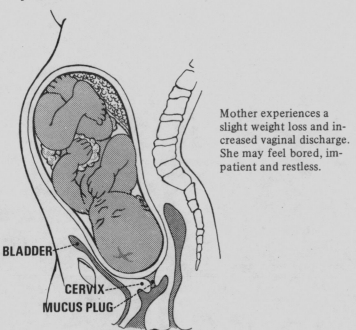

Mother experiences a slight weight loss and increased vaginal discharge. She may feel bored, impatient and restless.

BLADDER

CERVIX

MUCUS PLUG

False labor contractions may become so rhythmical and of such duration that the mother thinks she is in true labor. The following chart has been prepared to compare the contractions of false labor and true labor. When the mother thinks she is in true labor contact should be made with the physician or maternity staff. There should be no embarrassment in the event of mistaking false for true labor.

## COMPARISON OF TRUE AND FALSE LABOR CONTRACTIONS

| CONTRACTIONS | |
| --- | --- |
| FALSE LABOR | TRUE LABOR |
| Pain centered in back. | Pain in small of back extends to abdomen and groin. |
| Variable duration and severity at irregular intervals. | Increase in duration and severity which occurs at regular intervals. |
| Relieved or stopped by walking. | Intensity increased by walking. |
| Contractions stopped by sedative. | Contractions not stopped by mild sedative. |

During the period preceding labor the mother should conserve her energy for labor, practice exercises or labor rehearsal, and make final preparations for going to the hospital.

## Labor and Delivery:

Labor is a normal process by which the baby and placenta are delivered. It is described as a series of three stages by which the baby as well as the umbilical cord, membranes, fluid and placenta (afterbirth) are moved out of the uterus. Labor may be triggered off by the combination of a number of factors such as hormonal action, size and maturity of the fetus, volume of the uterus and condition of the cervix. No one really knows what causes labor to begin when it does — usually it starts about 40 weeks after the first day of the last normal menstrual period.

## First Stage of Labor

During the first stage of labor the cervix thins and shortens. This is called effacement.

The opening of the cervix stretches from a few millimetres to approximately 10 centimetres (the width of five fingers) to allow the baby to pass through. This stretching or opening up is called dilation. This stage is usually longer with a first baby and can last up to 32 hours but averages about 12 hours for the first baby and approximately 6 hours with other babies.

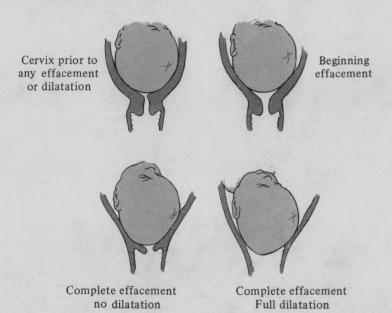

Cervix prior to any effacement or dilatation

Beginning effacement

Complete effacement
no dilatation

Complete effacement
Full dilatation

The following sections show what is happening, mother's reactions and what can be done during the early, active and transition phases of the first stage of labor. It may not be possible for the individual mother to tell when one phase stops and the next begins.

### Early Phase
The early phase is from the start of labor until the cervix opens to about 4 centimetres or dilation equal to the width of two fingers. It is the longest phase of the first stage of labor.

**What is Happening:**
- Contractions every 5-30 min. lasting 30-45 seconds.
- Backache and pelvic pressure.
- "Show" (slightly pinkish mucous discharge from the mucous plug in cervix comes out through the vagina).
- Rupture of membranes (may occur before labor begins or during 1st or 2nd stage).
- Cramps may resemble menstrual cramps.
- Or any combination of the above.

**Mother's Emotional Reactions:**
- Excited and relieved.
- Some apprehension.
- Sociable and talkative.
- Between contractions, impatient and eager for progress.

**Mother Can:**
- Notify doctor or have helper do so.
- Continue normal activity.
- Time contractions.
- Use breathing levels as needed.
- Eat a light meal (if physicians advises).
- Have a warm bath if someone is nearby and membranes have not ruptured.
- Lie on side using breathing levels and rock pelvis gently during contractions, or, kneel on bed, with head and arms on pillow doing exercises to relieve backache.

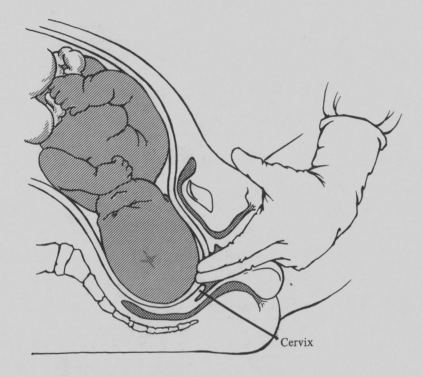

Cervix

**Helper Can:**
- Tell doctor about the strength, length and time between contraction (from start of one to start of next contraction).
- Help time frequency and duration of contraction by placing hand on abdomen.
- Encourage diversified normal activity.
- Check for relaxation.
- Give backrub if wanted.
- Offer support and encouragement.

## HYPERVENTILATION

**Hyperventilation** (overbreathing) may be caused by any type of rapid breathing when too much carbon dioxide is exhaled. The carbon dioxide level in the body regulates the brain in its control of breathing. If the low carbon dioxide tension causes the brain to withhold its stimulus to breathe, the patient may experience a "blackout" or fainting spell.

**Symptoms of hyperventilation include:**
1. Blurred vision,
2. Light-headedness, dizziness,
3. Tingling or numb hands and feet which may progress to cramps or muscle spasms.

**Hyperventilation can be prevented by:**
1. Keeping breathing shallow, in upper chest, throat and mouth.

**If hyperventilation does occur:**
1. Shallow breathing should be continued,
2. Breathing (especially exhaling) should be slowed down,
3. Breathing into and out of paper bag would help,
4. Breath can be held in full inspiration for a few seconds after contraction and before exhaling.

## Active Phase

The cervix dilates from 4 to 8 centimetres or the width of 4 fingers. This phase is shorter than the early phase.

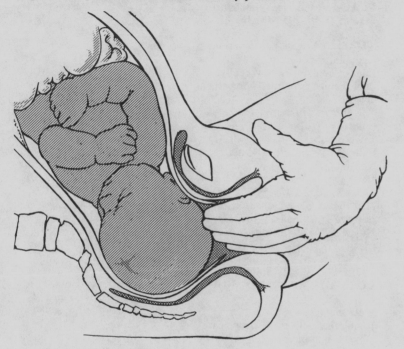

### What is Happening:
- This stage usually lasts 4-12 hours for first baby and up to 8 hours for subsequent babies.
- Increased, bloody show.
- Contractions every 3-5 min. lasting 45-60 seconds (becoming closer, stronger and of a longer duration).

### Mother's Emotional Reactions:
- Increasingly serious, quieter, pre-occupied with self and labor.
- Wants quiet companionship.
- May have ill-defined doubts, mother wonders if she can cope with contractions to come.
- Contractions are hard work, mother prefers not to talk or be distracted.

### Mother Can:
- Lie on side or if comfortable on back.
- Use breathing exercises as required.
- Relax and rest between contractions but remain alert.
- Concentrate on one contraction at a time.
- Take full, deep breaths before and after each contraction.
- If given an enema, expell it between contractions.

### Helper Can:
- Give frequent assurance, encouragement and coaching, and continuous companionship.
- Praise mother's efforts.
- Remind mother to urinate and to change position frequently.
- Wipe mother's face, neck and hands.
- Lightly stroke or massage (effleurage) abdomen during contractions, using talcum powder to help reduce friction.
- Watch for hyperventilation.

## Transition Phase

This is the shortest phase of the first stage. The cervix dilates from 8 to 10 centimetres during 5 to 20 contractions.

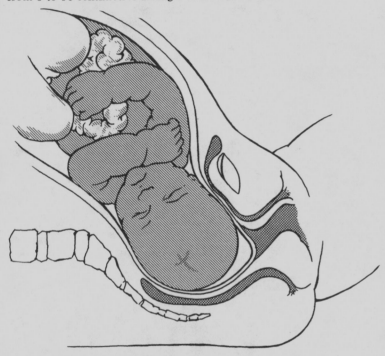

### What is Happening:
- Contractions every 2-3 minutes lasting 60-90 seconds — very strong and long (these contractions complete dilation).
- Show — heavy, dark and bloody.
- May have momentary nausea and vomiting, natural amnesia, leg cramps, trembling of extremities, backache, perspiration on forehead and around eyes.
- May feel hot or cold and restless.
- Relaxation is very difficult.
- Sleepy and drowsy between contractions.
- Rectal pressure — may feel an urge to push. DO NOT PUSH!!

### Mother's Emotional Reactions:
- Irritable, sensitive, short tempered.
- Cannot communicate verbally.
- May feel overwhelmed and want to give up.
- Bewildered, frustrated and temporarily discouraged.
- Exhausted.
- Cannot bear to be left alone.
- Considerable difficulty concentrating and relaxing during and between contractions.
- May feel surprised, overwhelmed or even frightened at urge to push.
- May speak with hostility to team.

### Mother Can:
- Use transition breathing. DO NOT PUSH! DO NOT HOLD BREATH!
- Stay relaxed.
- Remember delivery is close now.
- Do not tighten anus, but let pelvic floor relax and let vagina bulge forward.

### Remind Mother:
- That this phase is short and later pushing will feel better.
- To blow out to prevent pushing.
- Birth is imminent.
- To change position (sit up with back support, knees apart, heels together).
- To keep eyes open and to concentrate.

### Helper Can:
- Stay with mother - she needs constant encouragement, coaching and reassurance of normalcy of sensations and progress.
- Give firm, positive guidance and continuous low key verbal coaching.
- Can help by breathing through each contraction with the mother.

## Second Stage of Labor

During the second stage of labor the baby is pushed out through the birth canal. This is the active, hardworking stage of labor, and seldom lasts longer than an hour. The cervix is now fully open.

The baby usually faces the mother's spine flexing and extending its soft head to rotate around the pubic bone. The vagina easily stretches to allow the baby to pass through as shown in the picture opposite.

### What is Happening:
- Contractions every 2-3 minutes lasting 60-90 seconds are powerful, expulsive in nature, but further apart. Irresistable urge to push (pushing usually feels good if perineum is relaxed and the mother works with urge to push).
- Rectal bulging — backache stops.
- As head moves down birth canal, there is groin pressure, splitting sensation, and a burning feeling. May feel baby is "stuck".
- As baby's head crowns, doctor will order mother to stop pushing.
- Head is born, then shoulders; the rest of the baby slips out easily.

### Mother's Emotional Reactions:
- Surprised, overwhelmed or frightened by pushing sensation.
- Very tired but a revival of determination and burst of energy.
- Pressure on rectum may cause anxiety and hesitation to push.
- Drowsy and peaceful between contractions.
- Self-concern, indifferent to surroundings, excited, absorbed, impatient for progress.
- Mental alertness and excitement replaces drowsiness and discouragement.

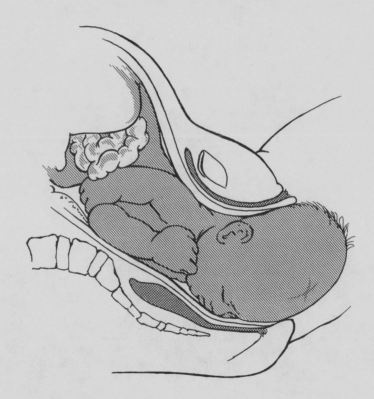

**Mother Can:**
- Put chin on chest and tongue on roof of mouth or just relax tongue.
- Put legs up on supports (stirrups) or mother may support legs herself.
- Bend elbows and grip legs with hands or hold hand grips.
- Relax pelvic muscles.
- Hold breath and push with contractions.
- Rest back gently when contractions finish.
- Breathe as instructed, pant if requested.

**Helper Can:**
- Coach with each contraction.
- Adjust mirror near end of delivery table if mother wishes to watch baby being born.

**Remind mother:**
- To relax her perineum.
- Pant when doctor says to stop pushing.
- Look in mirror.
- Take deep, full breaths.
- Rest fully between contractions.
- Tell her when head is visible and describe progress.
- Praise her accomplishment.

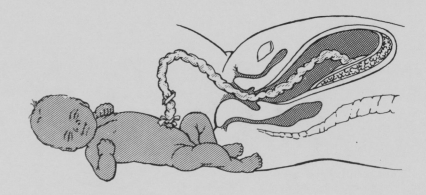

**NOTES**

The doctor may make a cut at the opening of the vagina, under a local anaesthetic, to enlarge the opening. This is called an *episiotomy* which will be stitched after delivery. It allows the baby's head to be born more easily and prevents any tearing of the maternal tissues. The doctor places clamps on the umbilical cord and cuts it to separate baby from the placenta.

## Third Stage of Labor

During the last stage of labor the uterus contracts to become smaller and the placenta completes its separation from the lining of the uterus.

### What is Happening:

- Contractions temporarily cease after birth and may resume.
- Uterus rises in abdomen and takes globular shape (grapefruit size).
- The uterus contracts to expel the placenta in 5-20 minutes.
- A gush of blood may precede or accompany expulsion of placenta.
- Doctor or nurse may push on abdomen to aid expulsion.
- Oxytocin injection to contract uterus.
- Episiotomy repaired under local anaesthetic.

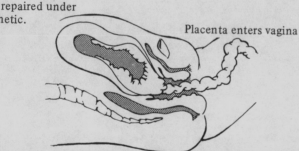
Placenta begins to separate

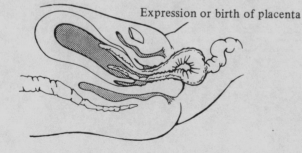
Placenta enters vagina

Expression or birth of placenta

### Mother's Initial Reaction:

- Euphoria, pure ecstasy is common; relief, gratitude, disbelief, wonder, joy, excitement. (Although some mothers don't experience any particular feeling).
- Exhausted, but often too excited to notice.
- PRIDE AND FULFILLMENT.
- Ravenously hungry and thirsty.
- Focuses on baby and seeks reassurance that baby is normal.
- May be sleepy when excitement subsides, or so excited that she is unable to sleep.
- Often unaware of placenta expulsion or episiotomy repair.

### Mother Can:

- Remain relaxed and push gently if asked.
- Lie back and enjoy baby with partner, remembering how important it is to keep baby warm.
- Allow baby to suckle (as soon as physician approves).

### Helper Can:

- Praise mother's accomplishment.
- Reassure mother about baby's condition.
- Remind her that a heated crib and suctioning of the baby are routine procedures.
- Ask if mother may have nourishment.
- Ask physician for permission to hold baby.

## The Newborn Baby :

The reward of pregnancy and labor is the newborn baby, and so it seems important to give parents a description about how the baby looks at first as seen by other new parents. One father, who was not present for his baby's birth, recalled his baby as looking like a "wrinkled prune" when first seen.

In reviewing the reactions of fathers who watched their babies being born, it was noted that they mentioned frequently the sex of the baby and the change in the baby's color from a darkish color to pink. The warmth of the baby's body when held was also a surprise. The fathers described their own emotional reaction and feelings of joy and pride in seeing the baby born rather than the physical appearance of the baby.

The newborn baby on the average weighs about 3,300 grams (7 lbs.) and is 58 cm (20") in length. The five senses: vision, hearing, feeling, taste and smell are present although not fully developed.

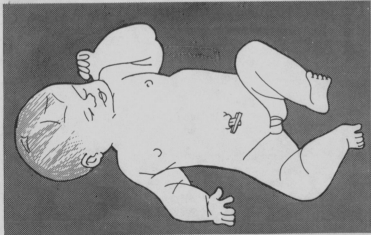

The head, as shown in picture above, is very large by adult standards in proportion to the rest of his body. His arms and legs are short and his bones are soft. His muscles are still soft and flabby, but he puts them to work at once wriggling and squirming. His skin may be red and mottled and is usually covered with a whitish creamy substance called vernix.

The baby's head may seem misshapen especially if labor has been long as the bones of the head mold and adjust themselves to provide for an easier delivery. The soft spot on the top of the baby's head is covered by a tough membrane. This spot is called a fontanel and closes in generally by 12 to 18 months of age. Parents sometimes worry about this spot but there is very little risk of hurting the baby there.

After baby's breathing has been well established and the cord is clamped and cut, the baby is dried with a towel or blanket and is ready to be held by the father and to be put to the mother's breast.

## NOTES

# NOTES

CHAPTER 7

## AFTER THE BIRTH

The first hours after the birth are a special time. Bonding is promoted if the newborn and mother are close to each other during baby's first period of alertness, and to begin suckling unless for some reason this is not wanted or possible. Father, too, wants to touch, hold and cuddle his new son or daughter.

Over the next few days both parents also need time to review what has happened, to discuss details of labor and delivery and to decide on questions they want to ask their physician and nurses.

In this section, some of the procedures, routines and current thinking about the immediate postpartum are presented with the hope that parents will discuss these topics with each other, their physician, in prenatal classes and during the hospital tour.

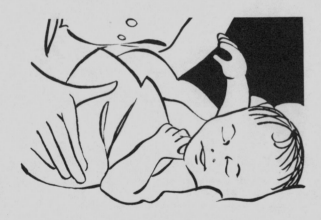

**The Newborn:**

### Apgar Score

Most babies of normal pregnancy and uncomplicated labor will breathe spontaneously, be active and crying, and within one or two minutes have a pink coloring. Their condition and adaptation to independent existence are assessed at one and five minutes after birth using a special scoring system developed by Dr. Virginia Apgar which takes into account heart rate, breathing activity, color, muscle tone and reflex reactions.

### Suctioning

Routinely, all babies are suctioned to remove any mucus or fluid from the throat and upper airway. If a baby should require resuscitation, equipment and medications are immediately available in the delivery room.

### Cord Care

Soon after birth the umbilical cord is clamped and cut, then an antiseptic and drying agent such as alcohol or triple dye (a purple dye) is applied. Over the next one to three weeks, or occasionally longer, the moist, soft cord dries up into a dark little stump and falls off. During that time it is important to give cord care as described in the baby bath part of this book or according to the instructions given by the hospital nursery staff when a mother and baby are discharged. If questions or worries arise at home parents should phone their physician for advice.

### Keeping Baby Warm

With skin still wet from the watery surroundings of the uterus, the newborn can quickly lose more than the usual amount of body heat through evaporation. For this reason the baby is immediately dried and wrapped in warm towels or placed under a special lamp. It is known that extreme heat loss causes "cold stress" which is especially serious for premature babies and infants who have required resuscitation.

## Care of Eyes with Silver Nitrate

Because there is a high prevalence of gonorrhea and a woman may not know that she is infected, B.C. law requires that a few drops of a 1% solution of silver nitrate be placed in all newborns' eyes. This is done to prevent blindness as a result of infection from any gonorrheal organisms that may have been encountered by the baby on the way through the birth canal.

Silver nitrate is the recommended treatment mainly because it is the only known drug to effectively prevent the infection.

## Screening Tests for Inborn Errors of Metabolism

### Phenylketonuria (PKU)

By the fourth or fifth day after birth, a few drops of blood are taken from the baby's heel and mailed to a central laboratory to be tested for phenylketonuria (PKU). In this inherited disease, the baby lacks a liver enzyme required to metabolize phenylalanine, one of the common amino acids in protein foods such as milk. When phenylalanine is not processed properly, certain break-down products accumulate in the blood, which can lead to mental retardation unless the condition is detected and managed as early as possible. This condition only occurs once in every 18,000 live births.*

If the screening test is positive, more tests are carried out. If the diagnosis is confirmed, the baby's diet must be adjusted, to include a special milk substitute.

### Hypothyroidism

From the sample of blood taken for the PKU test, screening is also done for hypothyroidism. In this disease the thyroid gland is underactive and does not produce sufficient thyroid hormone for normal brain and body development. If undetected very early and untreated, it can result in severe mental retardation but is only found in one of every 8000 babies born.*

*Statistics for B.C. obtained from the Health Surveillance Registry, B.C. Ministry of Health, Victoria, B.C., 1979.

### Other "Inborn Errors"

A number of other inherited diseases can be detected through urinalysis screening. For these tests, mothers are given a kit when they leave hospital and are requested to forward a sample of the baby's urine to the laboratory after he is three weeks old.

## Circumcision

Circumcision, or removing the foreskin covering the tip of the male infant's penis, is still customary in some families, countries, and religious groups. When making a decision on this matter, parents will find that physicians are not agreed on whether circumcision is necessary as a routine procedure. Generally, however, modern thinking in North America and Britain is that there is no medical reason for circumcision of a newborn infant and that the problems of uncleanliness and infection that it was intended to prevent can also be avoided by everyday good hygiene. Parents should know that the Canadian Pediatric Society does *not* recommend routine circumcision.

If the baby is circumcised, a small strip of gauze covered with vaseline may be wrapped loosely around the end of the penis to prevent the diaper from sticking. This piece of gauze simply soaks off in a few days.

## Intensive Care Nursery

As either a separate unit or part of the regular nursery, the intensive care nursery is designed for premature, low birth-weight babies or infants who, for various reasons, need special observation and care. Although such care does require the baby to be apart from mother for varying intervals of time, both parents are encouraged to visit and take part in the care of their baby as often as possible. Specially trained nurses are present at all times to work with the pediatrician and family physician in giving the newborn every chance possible for a healthy start in life.

**The Mother:**

## Lochia (Flow)

Following the baby's birth there will be some bleeding and discharge from the vagina for the next two to six weeks as the uterus sheds and renews its lining. Over the first two to three days, this flow is dark with clots and has a fleshy odour, then lessens and becomes brownish, similar to the last days of a menstrual period. After the tenth day, the discharge is yellowish white. The mother should call the doctor or nurse if her flow differs very much from that described. He or she will want to know about the presence of clots, the number of pads used and if the flow is foul-smelling.

The nurses in hospital teach every mother how to give herself "peri-care" which is careful cleansing of the perineum to prevent infection and odor, to promote healing and for comfort. Although procedures differ from hospital to hospital, one way to do peri-care is as follows:

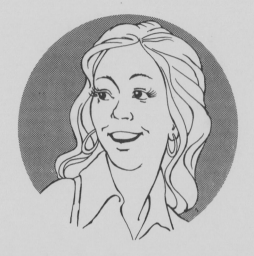

---

### PERI-CARE

i   *Wash hands* and have clean sanitary pad close to toilet.

ii   Fill a clean bowl with warm soapy water.

iii   Remove soiled sanitary pad.

iv   While sitting on toilet, pour the warm soapy water over perineum.

v   *Rinse* by pouring as many bowlfuls of warm water over perineum as needed.

vi   *Pat* with soft clean wipes from *front* to *back*.

vii   Put on new pad.

viii   Wrap and dispose of old pad.

ix   *Wash hands.*

x   Dry and put away bowl which is used *only for peri-care*.

---

## Menstruation

Often menstruation does not occur as long as the mother is breast-feeding, but this is not a certainty. If mother does not breast-feed her infant, menstruation should return within eight weeks after birth.

## Elimination

### Urination (Voiding)

The nerves to the uterus, bladder and lower intestine are closely linked and so are affected by the stretching in this area during birth. As a result, for a short time after birth, the mother may lose the sensation that her bladder is full. For this reason, the nurse asks the mother to urinate at regular intervals whether the mother thinks she must go or not. This prevents the bladder from becoming too full. The sensation returns to the bladder in one or two days.

### Bowel Movement

Most mothers have a bowel movement by the third day after birth. To make bowel elimination less difficult, the diet should include coarse, fibrous foods that stimulate bowel action. Naturally laxative foods such as whole grains, bran, dried fruits (especially prunes and figs), fruits and juices are helpful.

Some mothers may find that they require the aid of a laxative or enema in re-establishing regular bowel habits. This would be ordered by the doctor.

*Hemorrhoids* can be a bother after birth as well as during pregnancy due to the greater pressure in blood vessels of the pelvis. This can result in swelling and protrusion of the veins of the anus and lower rectum, causing general discomfort, pain and some bleeding. Relief can be obtained by avoiding standing for long periods, keeping bowel movements soft to avoid straining when going to the bathroom, and use of special pads and ointments.

## Breasts and Nipples

### Engorgement
For two to three days after delivery the breasts secrete *colostrum* in increasing amounts. By the second or third day the breasts become engorged, firm, tense and tender as the blood and lymph (fluid) supply to the breasts increases. The degree of discomfort varies with each mother but lasts only 36-48 hours. Soon after the onset of this engorgement, the true milk is formed.

The breast-feeding mother can avoid much of the discomfort by nursing the baby before the breast begins to feel full and emptying the breast manually when the baby has had enough. The breast-feeding mother will also obtain relief by use of a good supporting bra, hot packs or ice packs and perhaps a pain reliever.

When the baby is having difficulty grasping the nipple due to fullness of the breast, a warm shower for mother and expressing a few drops before nursing will help. Some mothers find a breast shield helpful.

Once the let down reflex occurs and the milk comes in it may come too fast for the baby to swallow. This can be prevented by expressing a little before starting to nurse.

The mother who is not breast-feeding must avoid any stimulation of milk formation by *not* massaging, pumping or allowing hot showers to fall on the breasts or nipples. A medication to suppress milk formation is usually effective but the relief may not be obtained until the engorgement subsides on it's own. Application of ice packs, a good supportive bra or binder, and a mild pain relieving medication will be helpful.

### Sore and Cracked Nipples
Sore nipples can be avoided usually by strengthening and softening them during pregnancy as described on page 37. However, some women, especially fair-skinned blondes and redheads, still experience some soreness of the nipples which begins around the twentieth feed, gets worse for 24-48 hours, then rapidly disappears. There are a number of measures to either prevent or alleviate the discomfort, if it occurs:

*The nipple should be kept dry.*

The nipples should be exposed to the air as much as possible by leaving bra flaps down, blowing gently with a hair drier or inserting small tea strainers in the bra cups. Reuseable or disposable pads placed in the bra should be changed frequently. Soft, washable cotton such as terry towelling, handkerchiefs and cut-up diapers or sanitary pads can be substituted for the commercially made breast pads. Plastic linings should be avoided since they hold in warmth and moisture, leading to irritation of the nipples. Sitting with the nipple 18 inches from a 20-25 watt light bulb for 5-10 minutes each day promotes healing. Sun lamps or exposure to sunlight is sometimes recommended but care must be taken to avoid sunburn. The doctor should be consulted about length of exposure to sun and also about pain relieving medication if required.

*Mother should avoid applying any substances that irritate the nipples.*

Only warm water should be used for cleaning the nipples. A wad of cotton may feel better than a face cloth but soap, tincture of benzoin, vaseline, alcohol or any other irritating substances should be avoided. Lanolin is recommended and should be rubbed well in to avoid blocking of ducts.

*Breast-feeding should not be stopped.*

Breast-feeding should continue so that the breasts don't overfill. It is important for baby to take the entire areola into his mouth, not just the nipple.

It is important for the mother to position herself so that the baby's mouth is at the same level as the breast so that the baby is not pulling down on the nipples. This means lying down to nurse or having pillows under baby if mother is sitting up.

To prevent nipples from becoming sore, baby's sucking should be limited to five minutes a side for the first few feeds then gradually increased in time. (If the nipples are very sore, taking an analgesic twenty minutes ahead of feeding time then limiting nursing to five minutes a side will help.) A pacifier may be used if baby needs more sucking time.

The less sore nipple should be used first so that the baby isn't as hungry and doesn't suck as hard on the second or sorer side. If both nipples are sore express some milk before beginning to nurse so that baby will not be sucking vigorously before the milk lets down.

In addition, changing mother's position as well as baby's position distributes the pressure to different areas of the nipple. The baby nurses more gently if fed more frequently. This may also help to prevent engorgement.

If the nipples are cracked the sight of blood from the nipple in the baby's mouth may alarm the mother but it will not hurt the baby. If white spots are noticed in the baby's mouth the doctor should be notified as sometimes the sore nipple is due to a fungus infection.

*It helps to relax when nursing.*

The mother should also try not to be tense as this prevents the milk from letting down and results in baby sucking more intensely.

After feeding baby, the breasts need to be dried and then a pure lanolin ointment may be used to keep the nipple soft. The lanolin should be massaged in well so that it does not keep the air from the nipples.

## Mastitis

Mastitis is an inflammation of the breasts that can develop whether the mother is breast-feeding or not. The mother may have a fever and chills as well as feeling generally sick and "achey". She may notice a reddened area on the breast, usually near the nipple, or a sore lump in the breast. The doctor should be contacted since antibiotics and pain relieving medication are frequently prescribed. A heating pad, hot water bottle or hot wet towel will be soothing. It is important for the mother to wear a good supporting bra and to get plenty of rest.

The mother who is breast-feeding will likely be encouraged to continue. Feedings should be started with the affected breast so that it is emptied. The feedings may have to be done for shorter periods of time but twice as often as usual to relieve breast tenderness.

If, for some reason, breast-feeding is stopped temporarily, the milk may be expressed manually so that the breast does not become engorged, and breast-feeding can be resumed.

Mother should refer to CHAPTER 8, Baby Feeding and Care, for detailed information on feeding by breast or bottle.

## Afterpains

After delivery the uterus contracts and descends into the pelvic area. These contractions are not usually felt after the first baby but may be painful for mothers who have had previous births, due to the repeated stretching of the uterine muscles which have lost some of their elasticity.

The contractions may be felt during breast-feeding as the sucking promotes uterine contractions.

Mothers can obtain relief by using the breathing and relaxation techniques learned at prenatal class. If the pains persist a mild pain relieving drug will be prescribed by the doctor.

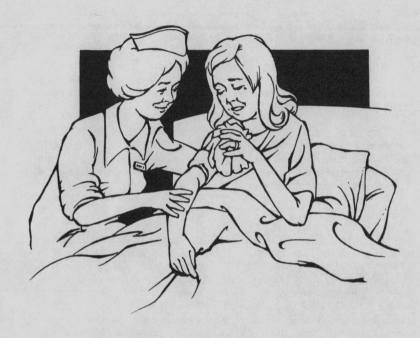

produce uneasiness. Where rooming-in is unavailable, some mothers feel anxious about being unable to see the baby when they want to. These emotions can be aggravated by the physical discomfort from the stitches, afterpains or sore breasts.

Mothers who feel like crying during this period should do so unashamedly as this may relieve the depression. It also helps to talk about these feelings with someone. Generally, the emotional distress will soon disappear as it is a normal reaction; but, if it persists, medical assistance may be needed.

## Rest

Once the excitement of the labor and delivery of the baby is complete the mother soon discovers how tired she is and may feel she needs a good sleep. Other mothers will find they are too elated to sleep.

A mother should take advantage of the short stay in the hospital and rest while she can. This is not always easy with the constant interruptions of a hospital routine so the relaxation techniques learned for labor may be useful at this time and later at home.

Although being up and about is encouraged in the hospital, this does not mean to be overly active. Sometimes mothers feel faint at first and so should make sure a chair is nearby when they get up.

## Nutrition

A mother's nutritional needs after the birth of a baby will depend on whether she breast-feeds or bottle-feeds her new infant. A breast-feeding mother should continue to eat the well-balanced diet consumed during pregnancy. Her calorie needs are even greater than during pregnancy. A breast-feeding mother's caloric needs are 500 calories /day greater than for a nonpregnant woman, including a new mother who chooses to bottle-feed her infant.

## Emotional Reactions

Within the first ten days after delivery some women experience temporary emotional distress frequently referred to as the "postpartum blues". As the term implies, the mother may feel restless, irritable, tearful, discouraged, depressed or helpless. This depressed mood may change abruptly to feelings of elation, being energetic and talkative.

There are both physical and emotional reasons for the mood changes. Sudden drops in estrogen and progesterone levels tend to contribute to them. Similar moods may have been experienced to a lesser degree, in the past, at the beginning of the menstrual period.

A mother who has never been a patient in hospital before may find the environment stressful. After all, the hospital staff and routines are unfamiliar, and being alone in a room or amongst strangers can

Foods should be selected from the Four Food Groups according to Canada's Food Guide which recommends:

Milk and Milk Products. . . . . . . . . . . . . . . . . . . . . . . 4 servings

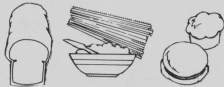

Bread and Cereals . . . . . . . . . . . . . . . . . . . . . . . . . . .3-5 servings

Meat and Alternates. . . . . . . . . . . . . . . . . . . . . . . . . 2 servings

Fruits and Vegetables. . . . . . . . . . . . . . . . . . . . . . . . .4-5 servings

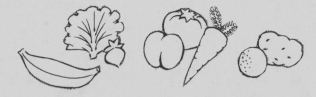

The additional calories required by a breast-feeding woman can be obtained by increasing the number and size of servings of foods from the Four Food Groups, or by adding fats and oils or other extras.

An average, healthy, breast-feeding mother with one infant requires approximately 2500 calories daily.

Breast-feeding women require more fluids than nonpregnant women. A breast-feeding woman should try to drink the equivalent of 8-10 glasses of fluid each day. Sources of fluids include milk, juice, water, soup, and ice cream.

The new mother who chooses to bottle-feed her infant should continue to eat according to Canada's Food Guide, while reducing her calorie intake back to her nonpregnant level. Canada's Food Guide will help the new mother to plan varied meals and to encourage good eating habits in new family members.

## Exercise

A regular exercise program to improve muscle tone and strength is a must for the new mother. These exercises are usually begun in hospital under the guidance of a doctor, physiotherapist or nurse then continued at home. Mothers may also take advantage of postnatal exercise programs offered by some health units and other agencies such as the "Y" (YM/YWCA). Programs differ, depending upon whether the baby was delivered vaginally or by Caesarian section, the mother's particular needs, and the preference of the physician, hospital and health unit. However, they all begin at a simple level, gently and slowly then gradually increase in frequency and strength. Good posture, whether standing, walking, or sitting is as important as it was during pregnancy. The muscles and joint structures need time to readjust to not carrying a baby. Correct posture avoids stress and pain.

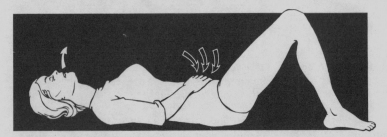

For most mothers, a daily walk with baby is pleasant and beneficial for both the exercise and the fresh air.

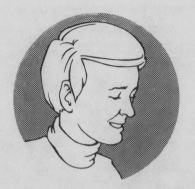

This is the time to present the children with a little gift from mother to baby, if one was brought to hospital for them. It is most important however, that they be reassured of mother's love and of their importance to her. They will want to hear that mother is pleased to see them.

If the children are unable to go to the hospital, telephone contact or messages sent home help them feel loved.

## Family Reactions:

### Father

The birth of a child is a joyful and inspiring event for father, but it also brings with it a troubling mixture of emotions that may include pride, concern, happiness, depression, jealousy, confidence or fear. This is a time when sharing of feelings between partners is so important.

The stresses father undergoes during the time of labor and delivery can leave him physically and emotionally drained.

So far he has been expected to play a supportive role to his wife as she undergoes major physiological and psychological changes. Yet his feelings are also important, and he will probably need emotional support and encouragement from time to time from his wife, friends and/or relatives. Frequently, father does not get an opportunity to express his true feelings and concerns after the birth as he becomes involved in the "passing-out-cigars" phase. All too frequently he is expected to assume the proud-father role and be the recipient of well-intentioned humor although he may not feel ready for it.

### Other Children

Many hospitals allow older children to visit mother after she has given birth to the new baby. This is a precious time for the children and should be arranged, if possible, when no other visitors will be present. They deserve mother's undivided attention first and foremost, before going to see the new baby.

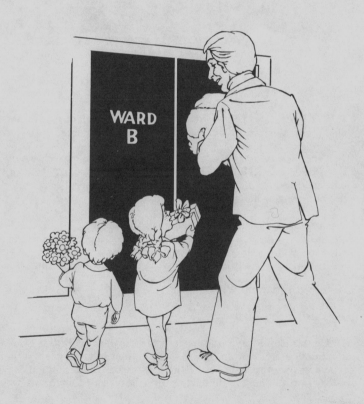

## Grandparents

Becoming a grandparent, especially for the first time, ushers in a new phase in life for the parents of the baby's mother and father. They are often proud and intrigued by their contribution to the baby's inheritance.

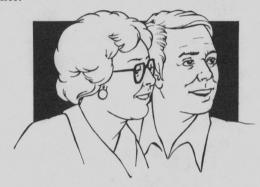

Grandparents sometimes see the baby as a second chance to parent, remembering the mistakes they made, or think they made.

Watching the grandchildren grow and mature provides new interests, goals and feelings of purpose for the grandparents. In turn, the memories recalled and passed on provide the new generation with a sense of belonging and pride in their heritage.

Sometimes the new parents may find coping with the small jealousies or hurt feelings that emerge between the two sets of parents difficult. Being able to communicate feelings openly and tactfully helps to forge a wonderful bond between the three generations.

## Legal and Financial Points:

### Registering the Birth

The birth of every child born in the province of British Columbia must be registered within 30 days. The father or mother is responsible for seeing that this is done. If the baby is born in a hospital, a registration form and help in filling it out will be provided by the staff.

If the child is born outside a hospital the parents get the forms from the District Registrar of Births, Deaths and Marriages in the local area.

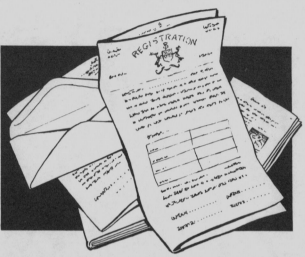

### Child of a Married Woman

In the eyes of the law the child of a legally married woman is the child of her husband and should be registered in his name. Exceptions to this, the forms to use, and procedure to follow are listed on the back of the birth registration form.

### Child of an Unmarried Woman

An unmarried woman registers the baby in her own name, but it may be registered in the father's name if *both* the father and mother make application and fill out an additional form. Any request for forms or inquiries regarding the registration of a birth should be directed to the District Registrar of Births, Deaths and Marriages.

### Some other points to note

The doctor who attended the birth is also required to send a notice of a live birth to the registrar following delivery. If the baby is born out of hospital the doctor should be asked to provide a statement. For people who live in an area where no doctor is available, this can be done by the public health nurse.

British Columbia does not allow parents to create a new hyphenated surname by joining the mother's and father's surnames with a hyphen. However, mother's maiden name can be used as an extra given name. This way it will still appear in the name, minus the hyphen.

When registering the baby's birth, parents can ask for copies of the *birth certificate*. This is needed for entry into the school system, for passport purposes and immigration, for a driver's licence and for marriage.

## Family Allowance

Once the baby's birth has been registered, an application can be made for Family Allowance. Hospitals have the forms, or they may be obtained from any post office. Payments begin in the month following the month of birth.

## Medical Services Coverage - doesn't occur automatically!

The hospital will provide every new mother with information about medical coverage in British Columbia. As a resident of British Columbia one of the parents is responsible for enrolling the new baby as a dependent on the family medical coverage.

If present medical coverage was obtained through the father's or mother's employer or union, they must be contacted to obtain medical coverage.

Parents covered through the Ministry of Human Resources must contact their social worker to obtain medical coverage for the baby.

For other parents who receive an individual billing and pay premiums directly to the Medical Services Plan, the hospital provides a form to send directly to the Medical Services Commission, B.C. Ministry of Health, in Victoria.

## CHAPTER 8

## BABY FEEDING AND CARE

### Feeding the Baby:

Feeding a baby is an easy and natural way of learning to mother a baby. Whether the decision is to breast-feed or bottle-feed the baby, feeding provides the baby with an opportunity to be held and become acquainted with a new person. Baby's most important need is tender, loving care in response to his gestures. During the early weeks especially, he needs to spend much of the day in mother's arms, enjoying the warmth and closeness of her body.

The decision to breast-feed or bottle-feed an infant has been discussed in CHAPTER 4. The practical management of breast-feeding and bottle-feeding follows.

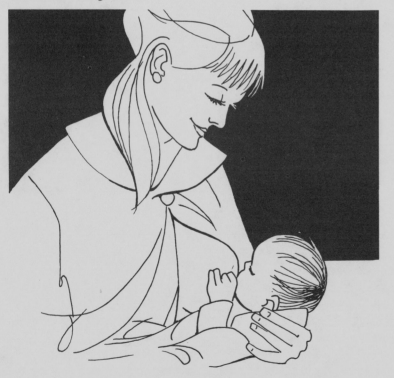

### Practical Management of Breast-Feeding

1. CLEANLINESS OF HANDS AND BREASTS is important. This helps protect the baby from infection. Hands should be washed with soap and water before each nursing. Clean water is sufficient for washing breasts as soap, antiseptics and various skin preparations can cause excessive drying of the nipples.

2. MOTHER NEEDS TO MAKE HERSELF COMFORTABLE and to be relaxed as she holds the baby with his head higher than his abdomen. Some mothers prefer to nurse while lying down. A mother who sits up to nurse may find a pillow under the baby helps to keep his mouth at breast level.

3. PRIVACY, if preferred, can be arranged either at home or in the hospital. The nurse or father can be asked for assistance in obtaining privacy.

4. THE BABY NEEDS HELP TO START NURSING. Gentle squeezing of the darker area around the nipple helps the baby get most of it into his mouth. After he starts to suck, the area can be released so that the milk flows freely. The baby should *not* have *just* the nipple in his mouth.

5. WHEN THE BREAST IS FULL AND FIRM the mother should use one finger to press the breast away from the baby's nose so that he can breathe while nursing.

6. EMPTYING THE BREASTS ADEQUATELY during the establishment of breast-feeding is important to avoid the discomfort of excess fullness. Uncomfortable fullness of the breasts can be prevented by nursing frequently for short periods of time at both breasts as soon as possible following birth. Nursing at each breast every 2 to 3 hours to empty colostrum stimulates milk yield.

7. BOTH BREASTS SHOULD BE TRIED AT EACH FEEDING although baby may not want to take the second breast. Five minutes on each side is usually long enough in the beginning and, if no soreness develops, the nursing time can be increased gradually to

10-15 minutes on each side.

8. NEW BABIES SOMETIMES FALL ASLEEP AFTER NURSING FROM THE FIRST BREAST. Changing his diaper will wake him up a little and then he will usually nurse himself to sleep on the second breast.

9. EACH FEEDING SHOULD BEGIN ON THE ALTERNATE BREAST. A safety pin on the brassiere strap can serve as a reminder about which breast to start with for the next feeding.

10. THE NIPPLE SHOULDN'T BE PULLED FROM THE BABY'S MOUTH as this causes the nipple to get sore. The suction can be broken by lifting up the corner of the baby's mouth with mother's little finger.

11. MOTHER SHOULD WELCOME THE BABY EVEN IF BROUGHT TO HER WHILE SHE IS SLEEPING as the night feedings help to bring the milk in quickly. There will be less swelling the sooner nursing begins.

12. WEARING A NURSING BRA provides comforting support and helps to keep the tissues from stretching. If the flap inside the bra sticks to the nipples it can be moistened before lowering to avoid breaking the skin. The flap should be dry before replacing it.

13. LEAVING THE FLAPS OF THE NURSING BRA DOWN for a while after nursing allows the nipples to be exposed to the air, helping to prevent sore nipples. Lanolin may be applied lightly after the nipples have dried sufficiently. Plastic linings should be removed from the brassiere so that the nipples get more air. Usually any tenderness will soon go away by itself.

14. CRAMPS ARE NOT UNUSUAL during early breast-feeding as this is nature's way of returning the uterus to its normal size.

15. THE LET DOWN REFLEX which allows the milk to flow from the production area of the breast to the nipple can be delayed by anxiety and tension. Therefore, it is important for mother to be relaxed and to enjoy nursing the baby. Rest, privacy, relaxation, patience and a positive attitude are important elements of successful breast-feeding.

16. BEING PATIENT helps, as the milk supply may take up to six weeks to become fully established. If a mother is worried about baby getting enough breast milk her physician or public health nurse may be called for advice.

17. ALTHOUGH BREAST MILK LOOKS THIN AND WATERY it is still the best food for the baby.

18. THE MILK SUPPLY IS NOT LOST AS THE BREASTS BECOME SMALLER AND MORE NORMAL IN SIZE. It only means that the swelling has gone down and the milk supply has adjusted to the baby's needs.

19. WHEN BREAST-FEEDING IS GOING WELL, THE BABY CAN BE GIVEN A BOTTLE WHEN MOTHER IS AWAY. It is advisable to leave only enough formula or breast milk to satisfy baby while mother is away.

20. IF MOTHER PLANS TO BE AWAY 6-8 HOURS, the milk can be expressed by hand or by breast pump to prevent the breasts from filling and caking. As soon as mother returns home, she will want to nurse her baby to relieve the fullness of her breasts.

21. VERY LOOSE STOOLS ARE NORMAL FOR A BREAST-FEEDING BABY. Some babies soil a diaper at each feeding. Other babies might go five or six days without a bowel movement — both are normal.

22. SIX OR MORE WET DIAPERS A DAY of pale urine indicates that the baby is getting enough fluid.

23. MOTHER NEEDS TO DRINK WATER FOR TWO. It is good to make a habit of drinking a glass of water, juice or milk before breast-feeding the baby. Ample fluids are important but there is no particular drink (or food) that makes a mother have more milk.

24. COMPANY, EXCITEMENT OR UPSETS SOMETIMES HOLD BACK THE FLOW OF BREAST MILK so the home surroundings should be arranged to minimize confusion for the next few feedings. Many mothers find breast-feeding comforting in times of stress.

25. AS MUCH REST AS POSSIBLE SHOULD BE OBTAINED IN THE FIRST FEW WEEKS. Mother gets off to a better start with breast-feeding if a nap is taken whenever possible, especially during the first two weeks.

26. LEAKING CAN BE STOPPED by pressing the palm of the hand against the nipple until the tingling sensation stops.

27. NO MEDICATION OR DRUG SHOULD BE TAKEN UNLESS PRESCRIBED BY A PHYSICIAN who has been told that the mother is breast-feeding.

28. BIRTH CONTROL PILLS SHOULD NOT BE TAKEN BY BREAST-FEEDING MOTHERS. The physician or public health nurse can be asked for information about child spacing.

29. THERE IS USUALLY NO REASON FOR MOTHERS WHO ARE BREAST-FEEDING TO GIVE UP ANY WHOLESOME FOOD. Occasionally, the baby may be bothered by something the mother ate, but it is not usually necessary to give up that food entirely.

30. SOLID FOODS SHOULD NOT BE RUSHED. Most babies have some fussy times during the day or evening that are not necessarily due to hunger. If solid foods are given too early, the baby will be less eager to suck.

31. BREAST-FEEDING CAN BE CONTINUED DURING THE MENSTRUAL PERIOD. The baby may be fussy at the beginning of mother's period but the nutritional quality of the breast milk does not change.

32. A WORKING MOTHER CAN BREAST-FEED. The baby can be breast-fed while the mother is at home and expressed milk or formula can be fed to the baby while mother is at work. The breasts may have to be pumped until they adjust to the new schedule.

33. BREAST MILK CAN BE STORED in the refrigerator in sterile bottles for 24 hours (breast pump and any other equipment in contact with the milk should also be sterilized). If milk is to be stored longer, it should be expressed into sterile bottles and frozen quickly at -12° to -17°C (0° - 10°F) in a deep freeze or separate refrigerator freezer. Freezing compartments inside the refrigerator are not cold enough. Only one day's milk should be frozen in one container. Collections of milk from several days should not be pooled and frozen together. It must be remembered that freezing does not sterilize contaminated milk. Refrigerated or frozen breast milk can be quickly warmed before feeding by placing the milk container in a saucepan of hot water. It is not necessary to pasteurize or boil the mother's milk before feeding the baby.

34. THE SLEEPY BABY. A very placid baby will sometimes sleep four or five hours at a time and does not seem very hungry at feeding times. If such a baby is not gaining weight, he needs more frequent feedings. The extra attention often perks the baby up and more frequent nursing increases mother's milk supply.

35. AROUND SIX WEEKS BABY'S APPETITE MAY TAKE A JUMP. Increased nursing for a few days will ensure mother's milk supply meets his needs. THE MORE BABY NURSES, THE MORE MILK WILL BE PRODUCED.

36. SOME BABIES NEED BURPING ESPECIALLY IN THE EARLY MONTHS. OTHERS NEVER NEED IT. A little gentle patting on his back when changing to the other breast and when he is through nursing will help him burp. If he falls asleep on the breasts, baby can be laid down without burping, preferably on his right side.

37. WEANING NEED NOT BE UNCOMFORTABLE WHEN IT IS DONE GRADUALLY. When it is time to wean the baby, formula can be offered in a bottle or cup in place of a breast-feeding. About every seven days another bottle or cup-feeding is offered in place of a breast-feeding until all breast-feedings have been replaced.

## Vitamins and Minerals for the Breast-Fed Infant

If the mother is eating an adequate diet, breast milk provides all the required nutrients in adequate amounts, with the exception of Vitamin D and possibly fluoride.

Infants and children under three years of age require 10 $\mu$g (400 I.U.) Vitamin D daily. The supplement should be started at birth and continued until the child is receiving that amount from dietary sources, e.g. fortified milk.

In areas with non-fluoridated water, fluoride supplements should be given to infants and children. Parents should consult with their dentist, family physician or public health nurse regarding the dosage, and when to begin fluoride drops or tablets.

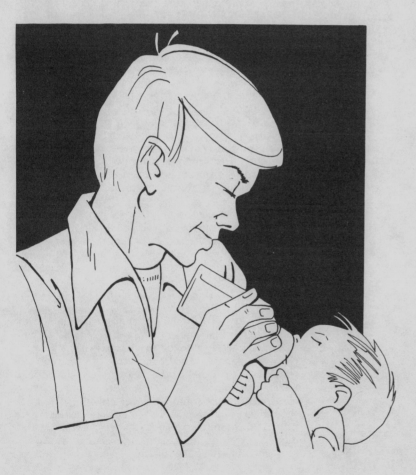

The drops or crushed and dissolved tablet may be placed directly on the baby's tongue or mixed with water or milk. Later, it may be mixed with his juice or food. Multiple vitamin and mineral supplements with fluoride are not recommended because of the difficulty of administering the correct dose of each nutrient.

## Practical Management of Bottle-Feeding

For parents, grandparents and babysitters, the following points will be helpful:

1. CLEANLINESS OF HANDS is important to help protect baby from infection. Hands should be washed with soap and water before each feeding.

2. MOTHER AND BABY NEED TO MAKE THEMSELVES COMFORTABLE AND RELAXED. Baby needs to be held with his head higher than his abdomen. Use of pillows often helps mother feel most comfortable.

3. BABY NEEDS TO FEEL MOTHER'S WARMTH AND CLOSENESS. Therefore, it is important for him to be cuddled and talked to gently as he is being fed. Another reason for holding the baby while bottle-feeding is to avoid any possibility of him choking.

4. BABY MAY NEED A LITTLE HELP when starting to feed from the bottle. The bottle should be held so that most of the rubber nipple is in the baby's mouth and at an angle so that milk fills the nipple and the baby does not swallow a large amount of air.

5. NEW BABIES SOMETIMES FALL ASLEEP WHILE FEEDING. Changing the diaper will waken the baby so that the feeding can continue until he falls asleep again, or the bottle is empty.

6. PULLING THE NIPPLE FROM THE BABY'S MOUTH MAY STARTLE HIM. The suction can be broken by gently lifting the corner of the baby's mouth with a finger.

7. BEING PATIENT WHILE FEEDING HELPS. Rushing a feeding causes anxiety in both the mother and baby. Company and excitement or upsets can interfere with a relaxed feeding.

8. SIX OR MORE WET DIAPERS A DAY of pale urine indicates that the baby is getting enough fluid.

9. BABY'S STOOLS VARY ACCORDING TO THE FORMULA. Babies who are on formula made from modified cow's milk have light yellow and firm stools which are passed once or twice daily. The composition of some commercially prepared formulas is so similar to that of breast milk that babies drinking these formulae have stools very like those of breast-fed babies (see page 85).

10. AS MUCH REST AS POSSIBLE SHOULD BE OBTAINED IN THE FIRST FEW WEEKS. Mother will be more relaxed and comfortable if she takes a nap whenever possible, especially during the first two weeks.

11. IT IS IMPORTANT TO BURP BABY half way through and at the end of each feeding by placing him over mother's shoulder or lap and patting his back gently. Lying him on his right side after a feeding will aid digestion, especially if he burps reluctantly or has a tendency to spit up.

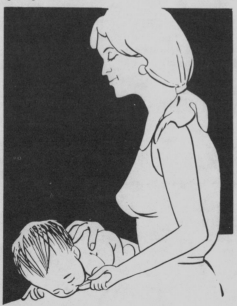

12. SOLID FOODS NEED NOT BE RUSHED. Most babies have some fussy times during the day or evening that are not necessarily due to hunger. If solid foods are given too early, the amount of milk consumed by the baby will be reduced and milk is the most important food for babies during the first six to twelve months.

## Preparation of Formula

The recommended method of formula preparation depends on the safety of the water supply, the type of equipment used, and the formula base. A method known as the aseptic method is most commonly used to prepare formula. This method involves the combining of clean water and formula ingredients in spotlessly clean equipment. No further sterilization of the formula is necessary.

1. Water — All formula prepared before an infant is six weeks old should be made with water which has been boiled vigorously for 2 minutes and then cooled. After the infant is six weeks old, and providing a safe municipal water supply is available, this step can be eliminated. When the water supply is from a well, or if the safety of the water is questioned, sterilization of the water should continue as long as the infant is on formula.

2. Equipment — Equipment which has been thoroughly washed with soap or detergent, rinsed well and air dried will have few remaining bacteria. It is important that all old formula or milk is removed with a brush. Particular attention should be made to cleaning the inside of bottles, nipples (water should be squeezed through nipple holes) and caps.

3. Formula — To make infant formula, an appropriate amount of cool water is first put into the clean container. Then the measured portion of formula powder, commercially prepared liquid concentrate or evaporated whole cow's milk plus a carbohydrate is added and mixed.
— Formulas must be diluted as per directions. Liquids should be measured carefully and level measures of powdered formula or carbohydrate used. Improperly diluted, overconcentrated formulas can cause serious problems in a young infant. NO CHANGES in

formula should be made without consulting the physician or public health nurse.

### Storage of Formula
Formula can be prepared by the single bottle as it is needed, or one day in advance. No more than a 24 hour supply of formula should be prepared at one time. In the event of inadequate refrigeration, single bottles should be prepared as they are needed.

All formula should be stored in the refrigerator at a temperature below 10°C (50°F). Open cans of formula or evaporated whole cow's milk should be kept tightly covered and refrigerated. Contents of these cans should be used within 24 hours of being opened.

### Temperature of Formula
Formulas may be served at room or body temperature depending upon the infant's preference. If the formula is to be warmed, the bottle of formula is heated in a saucepan with water or in an electric bottle warmer. Bottles should not be left out of the refrigerator to warm at room temperature as this gives bacteria an opportunity to grow.

Milk left over from one feeding should not be saved for the infant. It can very safely be used in preparing foods meant for older children or adults.

## Vitamins and Minerals for the Bottle-Fed Infant

Most commercial formulas contain adequate amounts of nutrients that are known to be required by an infant. The amounts of each nutrient in a particular formula preparation will be listed on the label.

In areas with non-fluoridated water, fluoride supplements should be given to infants and children. Parents should consult with their dentist, family physician or public health nurse regarding the dosage, and when to begin fluoride drops or tablets.

The drops or crushed and dissolved tablet may be placed directly on the baby's tongue or mixed with water or milk. Later, it may be mixed with his juice or food. Multiple vitamin and mineral supplements with fluoride are not recommended because of the difficulty of administering the correct dose of each nutrient.

For additional information on infant feeding, the booklet
Nutrition: DAY ONE to YEAR ONE
is available, free of charge, from the health unit.

## Bathing the Baby:

Ideally, bathing the baby should be a happy time, but this is not always so at first. Rooming-in, class instruction and helpful hints from many sources do not necessarily mean that parents can feel confident in performing that first memorable bath.

Although it is not a must for the baby to be bathed every day, the face, neck and bottom should always be washed daily, making sure that the skin folds are clean and dry.

For the first baby bath, a day should be picked when mother feels rested and if possible, father is home to help. The room should be warm, 22° - 27°C (72° - 80°F) and free from draft. After taking off any jewellery that might scratch baby, the parents should wash their hands then assemble the equipment as suggested on page 40 of CHAPTER 4.

The water for the bath should be about 37°C (98°F) or comfortably warm when tested with the mother's or father's elbow. If the bath is being done on a table, it should be a comfortable working height and protected with heavy plastic if not already waterproof. A blanket, pad or towel will provide a comfortable area for the baby.

The baby can be undressed in the crib and wrapped in a towel or blanket or left dressed until after the face and head are washed.

There are several ways to approach the actual bath:

- A SPONGE BATH can be given with baby lying on the pad on the table. This method is preferred by those who feel the baby should not be placed in the tub until the cord is off (navel healed).

- The baby's body can be lathered with soap and then placed in a LARGE BASIN for rinsing or the lathering can be done after the baby is placed in the basin. (If sink basin is used, it is important to run the cold water first so that the metal stopper does not become hot and burn baby. It is also important to protect baby from the protruding faucets.)

- Using the three-in-one approach, one parent can sit in the FAMILY BATH TUB and the baby can be passed to that parent for bathing. The baby will feel secure and probably cry less. When the bath is finished, the parent inside the bath passes baby to the parent outside the tub or if both parents were bathing, one parent steps out of the tub or gets out first to dry and clothe the baby.

## Face and Head

Bathing the baby is one job in which progress can be made by starting at the top and working down!

That means starting with baby's face by wiping it with a clean, warm facecloth *without soap*. There is no need to worry about doing anything further to the eyes, ears or nose unless there is discharge.

If there is discharge to be removed from the eyes, the wet corner of a clean facecloth or a piece of cotton should be used to wipe from the inner corner outwards. A clean corner or piece of cotton should be used for each eye.

When the ears need cleaning, the twisted end of a moist cloth or piece of cotton should be gently rotated in the outer part of the ear.

If the baby has a runny nose, it should be wiped and any crusting gently removed with a moist piece of cotton. Since this usually makes baby cry, it is just as well to leave the nose till the end of the bath.

From these comments, parents can see that it is unnecessary to probe inside of any of these openings with rigid cotton-tipped applicators as damage could be done to the delicate linings.

The baby's scalp can be washed by making a lather of soap on the hand or using shampoo. The baby is then picked up with one arm, using the hand to support the head. The soap can be rinsed off and the scalp and hair dried gently and thoroughly.

## Body, Arms and Legs

The baby feels more secure if he is spoken to reassuringly when being picked up and placed in the tub.

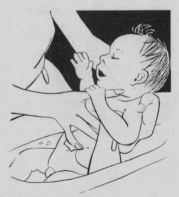

A firm hold, supporting the head, must be maintained. The soap is applied to the front and back of baby from his shoulders to his feet and then rinsed off well with the facecloth. The genital area is washed last. There is no need to push back and cleanse under the foreskin of baby boys who are uncircumcised. If baby has been circumcised, directions for care during the first days home should be obtained from the hospital staff.

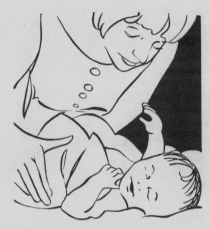

The baby is then lifted from the tub with the same hold and placed on the pad. The towel can be wrapped around him and then used to pat dry.

The skin folds and creases need to be dried well. It is not necessary to apply powder as sometimes perfumed powder can irritate the skin. As soon as the top is dried, the baby's shirt can be put on.

An absorbent ball (puff) can be used to dry around the genitals if necessary and wiping should be towards the anus. A fresh puff is used for each stroke. The groin area needs to be cleaned well and dried carefully to prevent irritation. Some mothers have found that dusting this area with a small amount of cornstarch on a puff helps to prevent chaffing. (Using a puff prevents the problem of powder getting into baby's nose and eyes.) The powder should be kept out of baby's reach and the puff used very carefully to avoid any chance of baby inhaling powder or cornstarch.

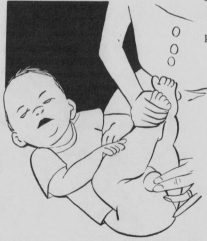

The diaper can then be put on and cord care given (until the navel heals). It is wise to place the baby's diaper below the navel to avoid irritation from a wet diaper.

## Cord Care

For many years the treatment of the stump of the umbilical cord was to avoid washing the area until the cord dropped off and the navel healed. This process usually took about two weeks. Sponging the area with alcohol on a sterile cotton swab was used to aid the healing by keeping the cord stump clean and dry.

This procedure is still used although many doctors now recommend cleansing the umbilical site well when baby is being bathed, then allowing the area to dry with or without the use of a drying agent. Leaving clothes off the area for periods of time also helps the drying process.

### Snug as a Bug in a Rug!

After baby has been bathed and cord care given, he will seem cozy if dressed in a gown or sleepers then wrapped snugly in a blanket. He usually enjoys having his hair brushed, but nails are better cut when he is asleep or at least sleepy.

Using these easy steps the baby's bath time can soon become a pleasant experience for the baby and the parents (after a few tries!).

## Safety for Baby:

"An ounce of prevention is worth a pound of cure" is an old adage but still very appropriate when considered in relation to accidents. As many accidents happen in the home, parents should be alert to factors that contribute to them at any time, but especially when a new life is dependent upon them.

The process of learning starts immediately for the newborn. He learns by touching, feeling, turning, reaching and experimenting, and as he is unable to recognize dangers himself, he must be protected from situations and objects that may harm him.

The baby's safety is not only the responsibility of the parent's but also of the children in the family, sitters and others who may be caring for him. The following are some preventive measures that can be taken according to the baby's stage of development.

A BABY IS COMPLETELY DEPENDENT ON OTHERS FOR HIS CARE. He should:

- never be left alone in his bath.

- always be kept in his crib, with the sides up, or in his baby carriage when he is not being handled.

- not be left alone with a toddler or a jealous pet.

- always be held to be fed as he may choke if left alone with his bottle propped.

- never be fed by someone who is smoking.

AT A SURPRISINGLY EARLY AGE HE WILL LEARN TO ROLL FROM SIDE TO SIDE. Therefore:

- the baby needs a crib with narrow spaces between the rungs so that the baby's head, arms or legs cannot become caught.

- he should never be left alone on a table, couch or bed.

- he should be placed in a playpen if he cannot be watched closely.

- the crib should be placed away from venetian blind cords.

- long cords on pacifiers should be avoided.

HE WILL LEARN TO MOVE HIS HAND TO HIS MOUTH AND WILL TRY TO EAT ANYTHING WITHIN REACH. Therefore:

- toys that are large and soft and have no removable parts are best.

- pins, needles, buttons, coins or marbles should be out of reach and kept in safe containers. Large safety pins, used for diapers should be closed when removed and placed out of reach.

- soothers or pacifiers should be large enough so as not to be swallowed and secure from breaking apart into smaller fragments. See page 42 for testing instructions.

- small objects should be kept out of the crib.

- plastic bags should be disposed of as they can cause suffocation.

- sharp objects, e.g. scissors, knives, forks, broken glass are potential hazards as are bones from fish or chicken.

HE WILL LEARN TO SIT UP, THEN TO CREEP, AND TO PULL HIMSELF TO HIS FEET, AND BEFORE LONG WILL START TO WALK. Therefore:

- guard rails or gates placed at the top and bottom of stairs protect against falls when baby starts to crawl. Ornaments, nuts or other objects that can be pulled off table tops need to be put away.

- cups of hot tea or coffee, pots on stoves, cords of tea kettles or percolators are best kept out of reach to avoid being pulled over.

- electrical outlets should be covered and extension cords disconnected. Safety outlets are essential.

In summary, the baby needs a place and space to exercise, to learn, and to roam; therefore, his environment should be "baby safe". Kitchens, bedrooms and bathrooms are usually the most dangerous rooms for babies. Household substances, medicines, cosmetics, hair sprays, sharp objects and scalding hot foods and liquids are hazards commonly found in these rooms.

Parents who check their homes may find many unsafe features that can cause accidents such as falls, poisonings, electrocutions, burns, cuts and gunshot wounds.

A knowledge of child development helps parents anticipate behavior that can lead to accidents. Planning to avoid these situations must always be uppermost in parents' minds. ACCIDENTS CAN BE PREVENTED.

Many very good pamphlets have been prepared on safety and can be obtained from the health unit. Information can also be obtained by writing to:

> The Canada Safety Council
> 1765 St. Laurent Blvd.
> Ottawa, Ontario
> K1G 3V4

## Common Concerns:

## Elimination

### Bowel Movements
THE APPEARANCE of the baby's bowel movement or stools changes every day in the first week.

From eight to 24 hours after birth the baby's first bowel movement is a sticky, odourless material which is greenish black to brownish green in color.

By the third to fifth day the stools are loose, contain mucus and are greenish yellow. Thereafter, the appearance depends on the type of feeding. Breast-fed babies have yellow, pasty stools. Frequency can vary from after every feeding to once every three to five days. Babies who are on formula made from modified cow's milk have light yellow and firm stools which are passed once or twice daily. The composition of some commercially prepared formula is so similar to that of breast milk that there may be little difference between the stools of these and breast-fed babies. When the baby starts to eat solids, his bowel movements will change to brown-colored, depending on the type of food eaten.

Parents should remember that newborns do grunt, get red in the face and grimace when passing stools. These normal pushing actions do not indicate constipation unless the stools are hard.

### Diarrhea (loose stools)
When baby has diarrhea, the stools become green, watery and foul smelling and may be expelled with considerable force. Baby's tummy may be distended and he may refuse feedings or even vomit. Diarrhea may be a symptom of infection in the baby's intestines usually caused by germs from his bottle, food or another person. Or, it may be the result of some other illness or irritation.

The baby should be given clear fluids only (boiled water if under six weeks of age) and the physician called if the diarrhea lasts more than a day.

### Constipation
Baby is constipated when his stools are hard. The frequency or regularity of bowel movements is not as important as their appearance. Steps should be taken to remedy the situation before baby's discomfort causes him to try to hold back the movement. Increasing fluid intake often helps correct constipation. If the baby is about three months or older and used to cereal, more fruit and vegetables, especially strained prunes or prune juice, will help soften the stools.

Constipation can be a sign that baby is not getting enough to eat, especially if he is crying right after a feeding or long before he should be hungry.

If constipation continues for more than a week or there is fresh blood in the baby's stools, the physician should be consulted. Laxatives and enemas should not be used unless suggested by the physician.

### Urination

Since the infant has urine in his bladder at birth, he may void or urinate immediately after birth or not for several hours. Because the kidneys are immature, the urine is dilute and a pink stain may be found on the diapers from the uric acid crystals found in the urine. Six or more wet diapers of pale urine in one day indicates that baby is getting enough to drink.

## Keeping the Baby the Right Temperature — Inside and Outdoors

Babies, like their parents, want to feel comfortably warm. This means an inside temperature of approximately 22°C (72°F) and no drafts. When the house is cooler, an extra sweater or booties would be in order. Because a baby does not perspire efficiently and can become dangerously overheated, an electric blanket, heating pad or hot water bottle should never be used. In summer, when temperatures soar, like his parents, he will enjoy being in his shirtsleeves.

There are many opinions about when baby should go outside. In deciding what to do, parents should keep in mind that baby's skin is very sensitive. For this reason and to avoid sunstroke, it is best in summer for baby to be kept in a cool, shady spot with eyes and head protected by a sunhat. In winter baby should be sheltered from moist, cold air which is apt to be chilling and a hood or bonnet put on baby when outside. In severe, cold weather parents are advised not to take babies out in the first month of life.

An important point to remember when protecting baby from the cold is to provide extra blankets below as well as on top of baby. The baby should be protected from intruding family pets and if insects are around, the carriage or basket should be covered with a fine netting.

Due to the diversity of climates in British Columbia as well as differing professional and cultural viewpoints on this topic, some parents may be interested in raising further points for discussion with their physician, public health nurse or at postnatal class.

## Colic

Colic generally begins after the second or third week of life and lasts until the third or fourth month, usually stopping quite suddenly. It is best described as a sudden abdominal pain which comes and goes and usually happens in the evening. The baby's abdomen feels hard and he draws up his knees and cries. What makes parents feel so helpless is that the loud and persistant cries continue even when the baby is lifted up and cuddled.

Although nobody knows what causes colic, it is possible that baby is hungry and needs more food or a different formula. More commonly, however, baby is probably being fed too often.

There is not much that can be done except for making certain that baby burps after meals, is kept warm and quiet, and is given plenty of cuddling. Lying baby across mother's or father's knee and gently rubbing his back may help relieve the gas in his intestines.

It is most difficult to keep calm while caring for a colicky baby. Parents will find that leaving baby with a trustworthy sitter and going out for an evening once in a while is a much needed help.

Parents are wise to consult their doctor rather than experiment with formula or medicines on their own.

## Hiccoughs

Many babies have frequent attacks of hiccoughs which are quite loud and explosive. They usually go away as the food digests in the stomach and really seem to bother parents more than baby. Sometimes a small drink of water or a change of position helps.

## Vomiting

Spitting up or regurgitation after a meal is very common and is not the same as vomiting. It is just getting rid of extra milk, and may be a sign of over-feeding or that baby has swallowed air and should be burped more often or that he has been moved about too actively following a meal.

If, however, the baby should begin to vomit, all solid food should be withheld and baby should be offered only water. If the water supply is unsafe or untested or if baby is under six weeks of age, the water should be boiled vigorously for two minutes, then cooled before giving to baby. Some physicians suggest adding 1 tbsp. of sugar or corn syrup to one half litre (approx. 1 pint) of water. If the vomiting continues, the physician should be consulted immediately.

## The Crying Baby

A certain amount of crying can be regarded as normal. Some babies cry because they are lonely and need a little cuddling to reassure them. Sometimes baby will be uncomfortable and need a change of position or a diaper change. A crying baby could be too hot or too cold.

Parents soon learn to understand what baby has in mind when he cries; a hungry cry is quite different from a sleepy cry or a cry of pain. Soon it is possible to tell when he is crying for attention, for very often a baby will cry for company, then stop and listen to see if somebody is coming, then start again a little louder. If it is bedtime and baby is in no discomfort, the best approach is a smile, a friendly word, perhaps a diaper change, a little caress and then leaving him.

## Diapers and Diaper Rash

One father, blessed with a sense of humor as well as a child, has written to the editors of this book about the parent-child relationship which centres around the function of diaper changing which he describes as the basis or bottom line of a dependent relationship. For, as this father explained, the diaper is a young child's environment. He lives in it, sleeps in it and openly does other things in it. It's the "other things" which parents have to learn to live with.

The old cotton or flannelette standby is no longer the only diaper available. A variety of disposable diapers are marketed and offer a convenience to the changer (and the washer!). In addition, there are both reuseable and disposable liners which may be used in conjunction with any diaper.

It is wise to compare the cost of different approaches to diapering (reuseable, disposable, diaper service), taking into account the initial cost, laundry and mother's time and health.

## Folding Diapers

There are a number of ways of folding diapers.

### Triangular Fold

For tiny babies the simplest method is to fold the diaper into a triangle and fasten the three corners in front with a single pin.

**TRIANGULAR FOLD**

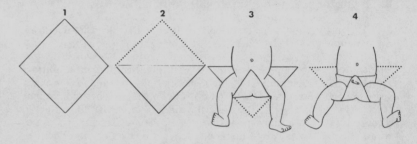

**KITE FOLD**

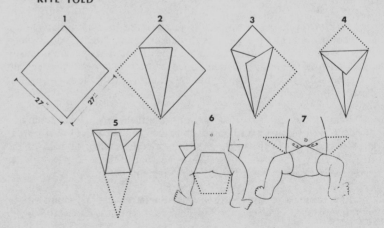

*Kite Fold*

To provide extra thickness at the back for a girl and at the front for a boy, a rectangular diaper can be folded into a square before folding the kite way.

One soon learns the signs, gestures and postures that indicate it's time to be "changed".

Some safety hints are to use only metal-headed diaper pins, never leaving them open or within the child's reach. Any time a pin is being pushed through the diaper, the changer's hand should be between the diaper and the baby to prevent striking the skin.

The baby should never be left unattended while being changed. Some people suggest changing them on a blanket on the floor.

**Diaper rash** is a general description of a number of skin conditions affecting baby's genital area. The rash is usually red and raw looking, varying in its severity. Most often it is due to the presence of ammonia formed by bacteria in the urine on the diapers, or the burning effect of a loose acidic bowel movement on the skin. Some diaper rashes can be of an allergic origin due to materials, soaps, powders or oils in contact with the skin. Less often it is due to a fungal infection. It is the rare child who has not experienced some diaper rash but the best cure is still prevention.

*To control diaper rash*, parents should take the appropriate action at the appropriate time. Diapers should be changed immediately when wet or soiled. The genital area should be cleansed with plain or soapy water and dried gently. It takes a lot of time to repeat these actions every time baby soils a diaper, but by doing so, half the battle against diaper rash is won.

Heat and air are also two very important factors. Heat encourages the bacteria to flourish and one of the more guilty parties is waterproof pants which trap in the urine or stools thus increasing the heat of the area. A good idea is to expose baby's bottom to the air for 15 minutes two or three times a day. This helps drying and healing.

For those who use cotton or flannelette diapers, laundering is very important. The cleaner the diapers — the less chance of diaper rash.

It is advisable to wash baby's diapers apart from other laundry, to use a mild soap and to rinse three times to ensure all soap is removed. In addition, parents will find the following helpful:

a) periodic boiling of diapers for 10 minutes after they have been washed and rinsed.

b) soaking diapers in a solution of vinegar and water (1 tbsp. vinegar and 3.5 litres (3 quarts) of water).

c) hanging the diapers in bright sunlight.

d) using a diaper liner.

There are many commercial cleaners, softeners and sterilizing compounds on the market but a cautious approach is best. Some of these chemicals may react with baby's skin.

**All the Other Questions Parents Have!**

Only some of the questions and concerns which new parents have about baby feeding and care have been covered in this chapter.

A list of child care books recommended by parents has been included in the section "Suggested Reading".

**NOTES**

# NOTES

# CHAPTER 9

## THE NEW FAMILY AT HOME

### Adapting to Parenthood:

THE MYTH OF PARENTHOOD is that once the baby arrives, everyone lives happily ever after. It's a lovely story, but it is really only a myth. The weeks after the baby's birth are a very sensitive time for the entire family. When mother and baby arrive home from the hospital, the parents suddenly find they are on their own with a totally dependent baby. Now the baby's needs have to be considered in all the family plans.

### Mother at Home

The mother may experience a mild depression after she gets home from hospital due to physical changes and to some emotional let-down after delivery (as discussed previously in CHAPTER 7). These feelings can be enhanced by trying to do everything right and not always succeeding. Becoming overtired and not receiving sufficient rest can also prolong the blues or let-down feelings.

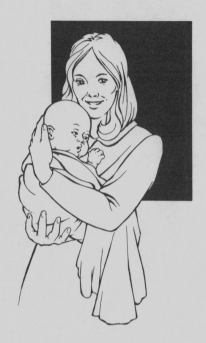

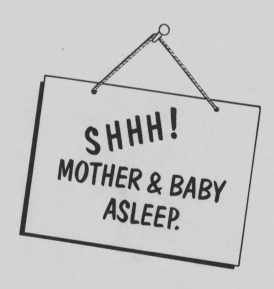

Too many visitors with well-meaning advice can also be a source of frustration to the new mother. A sign on the door can save the mother from uninvited guests and prevent interrupted rest breaks. It's important not to let guests interfere with mother's or baby's routines, especially in relation to interruption of rest periods. Mother shouldn't have to use her energy entertaining visitors and preparing food. Visitors can be invited to prepare a snack if they wish one but well placed signs can get messages across, in a non-verbal way and without loss of a friendship.

### Housekeeping

When a new mother comes home from the hospital, assistance with the housekeeping will help her regain her strength. If helpers are not available from within the family, the services of a homemaker can be used. The cost of the homemaker service is generally geared to family income.

A helper should be selected who can assist with preparing meals, taking phone calls and doing the cleaning. The mother's time should be spent enjoying and caring for the baby. Sometimes well-meaning helpers may want to reverse these roles, so mothers have to take care not to find themselves doing the housework while the helper enjoys the baby. When help is no longer available shortcuts can be taken to cut down on the mother's frustration.

Shortcuts such as tidying the beds while in the bedroom getting dressed for the day, piling the dishes in the sink and leaving them to soak, picking up the odds and ends that clutter the rooms and placing them in a big box helps keep the messy appearance away.

Two good books that provide practical suggestions on modern housekeeping are Karen Pryor's book on *Nursing Your Baby* and *Housekeeping Hints* by Heloise Cruise.

### Diaper Service
Many new mothers find a diaper service very useful, especially for the first few weeks. However, using a diaper service will depend upon the access to washing facilities, the availability of an adequate water supply for home laundry, and the cost of the diaper service and convenience.

Before the baby arrives, parents will want to check on the cost and details of the diaper service.

The provision of a diaper service for the new parents is one of the most acceptable gifts a friend or relative can provide.

### Father at Home
Learning to be a father is not necessarily easy, but with love, patience and understanding it can be enjoyable and rewarding. Sometimes during the adjustment stage it is forgotten that father may need help to adapt to his new role in life. It is important for him to be able to share his needs and feelings with his partner, as frequently this makes the marital relationship more secure.

If roles and responsibilities didn't change during pregnancy, most parents find they do in the postpartum. Besides re-allotment of house-hold tasks, money matters can be a concern for the new father. It is wise to consider budget adjustments carefully in advance of the baby's arrival and to keep expenses within reasonable limits. Additional financial items such as life insurance protection for the new family unit may need to be considered.

Father may also have to take the major role in making arrangements for a baby-sitter, so that he and his wife can go out together as this helps to renew their relationship and keep things in perspective when the baby's care seems to dominate so much of the mother's time.

It is important for fathers to realize that when it comes to infant care, they can be as capable as mothers.

### Friends
Some parents have found that getting to know other couples with young children is helpful. In this way mutual concerns can be discussed. Frequently, friendships develop among the couples who attend the same prenatal and postnatal classes.

Having a neighbor, relative or friend to help with the baby can provide relief for the parents. Support and guidance from someone with experience is helpful.

Upheavals within the household such as redecorating or moving just before or after the baby arrives should be avoided.

### Sitters
Parents should not feel trapped by the new addition to the family. Mothers, who feel they cannot leave the baby alone, may feel depressed and unhappy. Fathers also become restless and irritable.

After the baby arrives and mother has had a period to rest she should resume her social activities.

There are competent baby-sitters available in every community. If grandparents or relatives don't live nearby a check of the neighborhood may find an older neighbor who would appreciate being asked. In new suburbs, young couples can often arrange a baby-sitting co-operative to provide each other with some free time — usually this can be worked on a point system to be fair to all.

Reliable student sitters can usually be found by contacting the child care teacher or counsellor at a local high school, or the "Y" may give suggestions. There might also be a directory of sitters at a local community service centre or through church groups. It is important for parents to select sitters who have had adequate training. Sitters need to be given clear instructions to follow.

To find out more about resources in the community that can provide parents with help of various kinds, the local public health nurse can be contacted.

THE RESPONSIBILITIES OF PARENTHOOD MUST BE LEARNED — they are not natural instincts. It takes time for parents to learn their baby's ways, his eating habits, sleeping patterns, what his cries mean and how he can be comforted.

Most people learn their methods of raising a child from their parents. New parents should spend some time before the baby arrives talking about their ideas and finding out where they agree, and where they differ.

Both parents need not always agree on how to raise children, but after a thorough discussion, they should at least agree on a compromise. Children who have the love, attention and security they need when they are small, soon learn the differences in their parents' methods, and react accordingly, just as they will have to do with different people throughout their lives.

The most important thing to a new baby is to be loved. Holding, rocking, talking and singing to the baby will give him the sense of security he needs and also helps to develop trust in the adults providing care.

There are many good books available that provide guidance for parents in child raising. As well, the public health nurse can advise parents of the parenting groups available in each community.

### Brothers and Sisters
When a new baby arrives in a home where there are other children there are other adjustment problems. A young child in a family often has difficulty accepting the new baby, especially when the arrival often follows the first long separation of this child from mother. If he has been sent to a relative, or left with others while mother is in hospital, then returns to find her time almost totally occupied with the new person, little wonder he has intense feelings of jealously.

It is very important to reassure the other children that there is enough love and attention to go around. Sometimes parents have to make a point of directing the attention of visitors to the older child's activities and accomplishments — to make him realize he's still important.

The other children sometimes display forms of unusual behavior when too much attention is focused on the new baby. They may even revert to infant behavior (i.e., wetting, thumb sucking, crying, etc.) to gain attention. Recognizing these behaviors for what they are and giving the child some undivided time and attention can alleviate these behaviours.

Older children often appreciate being given some responsibility for the care of the baby — helping with baby's clothes, pushing the carriage, showing the baby to visitors, all help to make them feel that they are important in the family.

## Resuming Sexual Activity:

Traditionally, physicians have advised new mothers to wait until after the postpartum medical checkup before resuming sexual intercourse. Such advice was probably based on the fact that it takes 4-6 weeks for the body to return to its non-pregnant state. During this time the hormones and blood supply are readjusting, the uterus and vagina are returning to non-pregnant size, the perineum is recovering from stretching, bruising and possibly an episiotomy during childbirth and the mother's milk supply is either being established or repressed.

For most couples, however, it is not necessary to wait these 4-6 weeks and sexual intercourse can be resumed once the lochia is no longer red, any tears or the episiotomy have healed and the mother feels comfortable and rested (usually 1-2 weeks).

Therefore, it is important for parents to discuss this topic and birth control with the physician before going home from hospital.

There is considerable variation in patterns of sexual activity after childbirth depending upon when healing has taken place, how the woman feels from the physical and hormonal changes of the post-partum and both partners' interest in sex. In addition, there is the inevitable fatigue from the work of childbirth and baby's unpredictable feeding schedule — especially those nights!

It's not unusual for a woman to be disinterested in sexual activity for a while after baby's arrival — perhaps due to the hormonal changes and because she is so involved with the baby. Some husbands, too, have mixed feelings about sexual relations.

Breast-feeding doesn't prevent sexual response, but it does inhibit lubrication in the vagina. This lack of lubrication often occurs whether the mother is or isn't breast-feeding and a contraceptive or other appropriate water-soluable cream (not vaseline) is recommended. Normally, a woman who has been breast-feeding her infant may eject some milk from the breast during orgasm.

Once home, parents will find that what is most important is a true caring and sharing for both each other and the baby. With such understanding they will be able to discuss questions or problems. The physician and public health nurse are always willing to be contacted. As well, many new parents are finding that postnatal groups offer a supportive and enjoyable setting in which to exchange and help overcome concerns about sexual relations.

## Birth Control:

As mentioned in the previous section, it is important for new parents to discuss birth control methods with the physician before discharge from hospital since conception can occur in the first 4-6 weeks postpartum, even if the mother is breast-feeding.

The following chart is provided to summarize the various methods of birth control which a couple can consider.

Because the mother cannot be fitted for a diaphragm or IUD until 4-6 weeks postpartum and breast-feeding mothers are advised not to take the pill, alternate methods will have to be explored.

Information is available from - hospital class on family planning
- public health nurse's home visit
- physician
- postnatal classes at health unit
- family planning clinic

The final choice, of course, rests with the couple who best know what method suits their bodies, lifestyle and love-making.

## BIRTH CONTROL METHODS

## DIAPHRAGM WITH JELLY OR CREAM

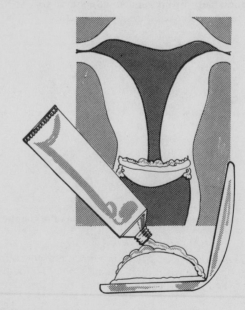

## Effectiveness:
With spermicidal jelly or cream — 2-3% failure; without spermicidal jelly or cream — 10-15% failure or higher.

## Description:
Thin, strong, flexible rubber shield which fits over the cervix.

Comes in different sizes.

Best if lubricated with a contraceptive jelly or cream (not foam which deteriorates rubber).

## Advantages:
Can't be felt by either partner.

## Disadvantages:
Can interfere with spontaneity of intercourse because of need to insert it first. Occasionally can be dislodged during intercourse.

## Special Instructions:
A *physician* must measure the woman before prescribing a diaphragm. He must also teach her to insert it correctly.

Diaphragm must be left in place for at least 8 hours after intercourse and can be left in for up to 24 hours.

After removal it should be washed and dried.

Douching is usually not necessary but if it is done, the diaphragm should be removed first.

A yearly check by the *doctor* is necessary to ensure diaphragm still fits. A change in size may also be needed *after having a baby* or following abortion, pelvic surgery and gain or loss of more than ten pounds.

# INTRAUTERINE DEVICE (IUD)
Different brands and designs, e.g. Loop, Coil, Shield.

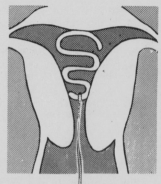

Copper T and 7 are most commonly used.

## Effectiveness:
2-5% failure rate.

## Description:
Small, flexible piece of sterile plastic which is inserted by the physician into the uterus.

Some IUD's are wrapped with a thin copper wire.

After simple insertion, the IUD is left in place for 2-3 years.

Doctor can remove IUD if a pregnancy is desired.

How IUD actually works is not fully understood but it appears to prevent the egg from implanting in the uterus.

## Advantages:
Continuous protection therefore nothing to remember or to interfere with spontaneity of intercourse. Sexual response may be improved because neither partner worries about possible pregnancy.

## Disadvantages:
Some women experience cramps during and after insertion. For a while, menstrual periods may be heavier with slight bleeding between periods. Occasionally device slips out unnoticed. IUD thread may be

felt by man during intercourse. Rare complications of infection and of IUD slipping through uterine wall into abdomen (surgery necessary).

## Special Instructions:
*Doctor* will recommend shape and size of IUD which best suits and fits uterus. Inserted during menstrual period.

Fine thread hangs down from IUD so woman can check that it is still in place by feeling with her fingers. Important to note either lengthening or absence of thread.

Thread is not in way of tampons during menstruation.

*After Childbirth* - best to wait until uterus returns to pre-pregnant state before fitting and insertion of IUD.

---

## CONDOM (rubber, safe, prophylactic)

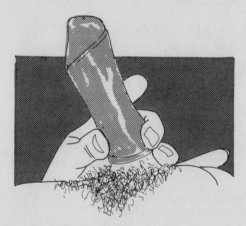

**Effectiveness:**
15-35% failure.

Risk of pregnancy is less if woman also uses a contraceptive cream, jelly or foam.

## Description:
Thin sheath rolled on and over the penis when it is erect.

Condoms may be dry or lubricated and come in different shapes, colour and textures.

A space with no air inside is left at the tip of the condom to catch the seminal fluid (sperm and semen) and prevent its escape into the vagina.

## Advantages:
No side effects. Readily available when needed. Can be bought at a drugstore without a prescription. Provides protection against venereal disease.

## Disadvantages:
Need to interrupt foreplay to put on condom. Can interfere with sensation.

## Special Instructions:
Since sperm can be released before climax, delay in putting on condom could result in pregnancy.

If the condom isn't made with a "balloon tip" care should be taken to leave a space at the end for the seminal fluid.

Slippage and leakage can be avoided if the man holds the condom in place as his penis becomes soft and if he withdraws promptly after ejaculation.

If disposable type, new condom should be used each time man has intercourse.

If a washable, reusable type is used, it must be washed and then checked for deterioration each time by blowing in it or filling it with water.

Condoms are frequently used for one month after woman begins the pill.

## VAGINAL FOAMS, CREAMS, JELLIES AND TABLETS

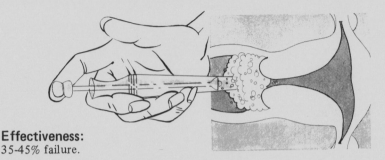

**Effectiveness:**
35-45% failure.

Foam, cream, jelly or tablet + condom is almost 100% *effective*.

**Description:**
Chemical barriers to kill and prevent sperm from entering the uterus.

**Advantages:**
Can't be felt when used except for their extra moisture. Can be bought at a drugstore without a prescription.

**Disadvantages:**
Must read label carefully. Similar feminine hygiene products on the market don't have the word CONTRACEPTIVE on their labels. Interferes with spontaneity of intercourse.

**Special Instructions:**
Because some women and men react differently to different preparations, it is wise to consult a *physician* before purchasing, but . . . better to use and ask after than not to use at all!

Care should be taken to insert the applicator as deep as possible into the vagina so cervix is covered with foam, cream or jelly.

Since foam container can become empty without much warning it is advisable to keep a second container in reserve.

Tablets take 10-15 minutes to dissolve before they are effective.

## ORAL CONTRACEPTIVE
"The Pill"

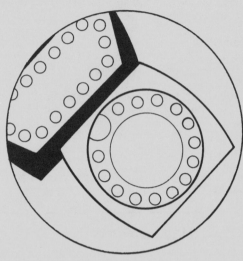

Dosage and type of pill decided upon by the physician.

**Effectiveness:**
Nearly 100% effective. Will not be effective if 2 days missed or taken "now and then".

**Description:**
Hormones in the pill prevent the monthly release of the woman's egg. No egg = no pregnancy.

**Advantages:**
Menstrual flow lighter and shorter usually.
Doesn't matter when or how often woman makes love: continuous protection.

## Disadvantages:

For first month or two some women develop pregnancy-like symptoms, e.g., nausea, tender breasts, chloasma (pregnancy mask), headaches, weight gain.

## Special Instructions:

Must be prescribed by a *physician*. Instructions on package must be followed carefully.

*Must not be taken if breast-feeding.*

If woman decides to get pregnant she should stop the pill at the end of the cycle then wait two or three months or re-establish menstrual cycle before getting pregnant.

Doctor will advise some women not to take the pill. Important to have a medical check-up since there are contraindications.
  breast-feeding
  blood clots or inflammation in veins
  serious liver disease
  cancer of breast or uterus

*May also be contraindicated for women who have or have had:*
  heart disease
  kidney disease
  high blood pressure
  diabetes
  epilepsy
  breast cysts
  fibroids of uterus
  migraine headaches
  severe mental depression
  sickle cell anemia
  gall bladder disease
  asthma
  smoking habit

## BREAST-FEEDING TO SPACE BABIES
(May be referred to as natural family planning).

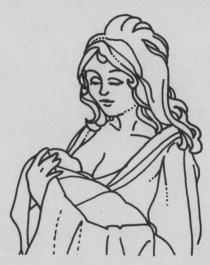

## Effectiveness:

Different studies report rates ranging from 100% successful to 9 pregnancies per 100 women using the method if *instructions followed for complete breast-feeding*. Not a reliable method for many of today's women. *Another method of birth control is advised*.

## Description:

Ovarian function is depressed during lactation probably due to the infant sucking.

Decrease in the frequency of breast-feeding or cessation of nursing results in re-establishment of ovarian function and reappearance of menstruation and ability to conceive.

## Advantages:

Lifestyle of "where mother goes, baby goes" appeals to many women and couples.
Inexpensive.

## Disadvantages:

Complete breast-feeding is difficult for the working mother and interrups some people's social lives.

## Special Instructions:

To successfully prevent conception through nursing means a mother must practice total or complete breast-feeding; that is:

- Baby should stay at breast a little longer even though nutritionally satisfied.

- Baby should be fed on demand.

- Mother should feed baby at all feedings, including nighttime. This means taking baby along on most outings and having baby sleep near enough to mother that night feeding is as easy as possible. If mother is away for a feeding, extra nursing when she returns is essential. Baby is usually willing to oblige.

- Baby should not be given solids before six months and then given finger foods.

- Baby should wait nine or more months before taking other liquids, unless he wants a cup. (Bottle-feeding, pacifiers, and even cups reduce amount of breast-feeding).

Very occasionally, mother may express milk to be used when she is away but she should be aware that even this brief absence from nursing may hasten return to fertility.

## WITHDRAWAL
### (Being careful)

35-40% failure.

## Effectiveness:

Failures occur often because of poor control or because some sperm may be discharged prior to ejaculation and may cause pregnancy.

## Description:

In this method the man withdraws his penis from inside the woman's vagina before the climax so the sperm aren't left in or near her body.

## Disadvantages:

Man or woman or both are frustrated because they are left unsatisfied sexually. Difficult to have the willpower to withdraw.

## Special Instructions :

Takes mutual motivation, willpower and co-operation.

## VASECTOMY (Male sterilization)

This is more a method of *planning no more family*.

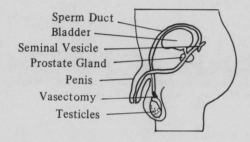

Sperm Duct
Bladder
Seminal Vesicle
Prostate Gland
Penis
Vasectomy
Testicles

### Effectiveness:
Practically 100% effective.

### Description:
In a simple surgical procedure, the vas deferens (tubes that transport sperm from testes) are cut and tied. After a vasectomy the sperm continue to form but because they can't get through the blocked area, they disintegrate and are absorbed into the local circulation and excreted.

After the vasectomy there will be some bruising and general tenderness.

A vasectomy does not decrease sex drive or potency.

### Advantages:
Can improve the couple's sex life because there is no fear of pregnancy.

### Disadvantages:
Is *irreversible*. Couple could change their minds about wanting more children or couples may find different partners e.g., divorce, remarriage. Possibility of complications is the same as for any surgical procedure, i.e., infection, bleeding, unusual pain or swelling.

### Special Instructions:
Before considering a vasectomy the following questions should be asked and answered with a "yes":

1. Do both partners wish to limit their family to its present size?

2. Are other methods of contraception unacceptable or impractical?

3. Is the husband willing to take the risks of a vasectomy?
   These are:
   (a) A small chance of surgical complications, as with any minor surgery;
   (b) A small chance of failure of sterilizing effect, as shown by sperm tests after the operation, necessitating a second operation;
   (c) Living to regret having been sterilized should there be a change in marital, familial or personal circumstances.

4. Are both partners agreed that the husband is the better choice, even though the wife is agreeable to sterilization of herself?

Light duties may be resumed the next day but heavy work should be put off for a week or so.

As advised by *physician*, patient collects samples of seminal fluid which are tested for presence of sperm which may be present.

To avoid pregnancy, it is essential to continue another method of birth control until tests indicate absence of sperm.

# TUBAL LIGATION (Female sterilization)

This is really a method of *planning no more family*.

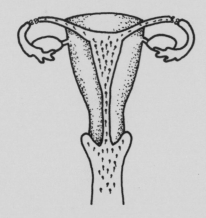

One of several surgical techniques may be used, such as:

1. abdominal incision – the doctor makes a small abdominal incision, then cuts and ties the Fallopian tubes.

2. laparoscopy – 1-2 tiny incisions made near umbilicus and metal tube inserted through which doctor can see and seal off Fallopian tubes.

3. vaginal – incision made at top of the vagina near the cervix then tubes cut and tied.

Practically 100% effective.

## Description:
The Fallopian tubes which carry the ripe egg from the ovary to the uterus each month are cut and tied or sealed off. This sterilizes the woman and makes her unable to become pregnant.

After the operation, the ovaries continue to release one egg a month which disintegrates at the end of the blocked-off tube as it had before in the uterus if not fertilized.

## Advantages:
Sexual pleasure may be increased because there is no fear of pregnancy.

## Disadvantages:
Is *irreversible*. Couple could change their minds about wanting more children or couples may find different partners e.g., divorce, remarriage. Possibility of complications is the same as for any surgical procedure, i.e., infection, bleeding, unusual pain or swelling.

## Special Instructions:
Before considering a tubal ligation the following questions should be asked and answered with a "yes":

1. Do both partners wish to limit their family to its present size?

2. Are other methods of contraception unacceptable or impractical?

3. Is the woman willing to take the risks of a tubal ligation?
   These are:
   (a) general anaesthesia;
   (b) a small chance of complications from abdominal surgery;
   (c) a small chance of failure of sterilization and the consequences of pregnancy;
   (d) living to regret having been sterilized should a child die or there be a change in marital circumstances.

4. Are both partners agreed that the woman is the better choice, even though a tubal ligation is a more complicated surgical procedure than a vasectomy?

Is effective immediately, therefore no need for any other form of birth control.

Sexual intercourse may not be resumed for six weeks if vaginal method of surgery was used.

# BASAL BODY TEMPERATURE METHOD (BBT)

May be referred to as natural family planning or rhythm method.

## Effectiveness:
Strict Method — .8% failure, Ricotta or Less Strict Method — 3.1% failure.

Providing couple follows instructions correctly. BECAUSE THIS IS DIFFICULT, A 15-30% FAILURE RATE IS MORE LIKELY.

## Description:
This method is based on the fact that the hormone, progesterone, is produced at the time of ovulation and causes a rise is body temperature.

By taking her temperature orally first thing in the morning after two-three hours of uninterrupted sleep (getting up to bathroom doesn't count), a woman can plot her not fertile "safe" and fertile "unsafe" days. Intercourse must be avoided on the "unsafe" days.

*Strict BBT Method*
Restricts intercourse to second safe period i.e., from third day after temperature rises to onset of menstruation.

*Ricotta or Less Strict BBT Method*
In addition to having intercourse from the third day after temperature rises to onset of menstruation, couple can have sexual relations for the first seven days of the woman's cycle if her cycle is more than 26 days long.

## Advantages:
Inexpensive.
No devices to spoil spontaneity of sex on the "safe" days. Even if other methods are preferred and used, it is useful to be able to fall back on this method in between other methods or after childbirth.

## Disadvantages:
Pits willpower versus passion on the "unsafe" days — requires firm commitment of both partners..
Not practical if poor marital relationship. Difficult to use for the woman who doesn't ovulate (some breast-feeding women), woman approaching menopause or one who has very long or very short periods.

## Special Instructions:
Partners must understand how the method works and co-operate in its use. There needs to be a loving relationship and mutual motivation to use the method.

SPECIFIC INSTRUCTIONS SHOULD BE OBTAINED IF THIS METHOD IS TO BE USED.

## OVULATION METHOD (Billings Method)

May be referred to as natural family planning or rhythm method.

### Effectiveness:
Different rates reported ranging from 100% effective to 5.4 pregnancies per 100 women using the method providing instructions followed.

As for the BBT method, a 15-30% failure rate is more realistic.

### Description:
The ovulation method is based on the fact that fertilization cannot occur without favorable cervical mucus. A woman assesses the consistency of her vaginal discharge each day to determine when ovulation is occurring. There is a particular recognizable mucous secretion when she is capable of conceiving. On these "unsafe" days she must not have sexual intercourse.

A chart with color-coded stamps is used to depict the mucous discharge.

### Advantages:
Useful in ovulating and unovulating women as well as menopausal and *lactating* mothers. Can also be successful when woman is discontinuing the pill and cycles are irregular. Useful method to fall back upon between other methods or after childbirth.
Inexpensive.
No devices to spoil spontaneity of sex on "safe" days.

### Disadvantages:
Cervicitis or vaginitis can reduce the effectiveness although some women can still "read their mucus". Pits willpower versus passion on the "unsafe" days. Requires firm commitment of both partners. Not practical if poor marital relationship.

### Special Instructions:
As for BBT, partners must understand how the method works and co-operate in its use. There needs to be a loving relationship and mutual motivation to use the method.

Must abstain from sexual relations for one month while establishing the method.

Instruction booklet by John Billings can be purchased at most bookstores. Individual or class instruction is required.

## SYMPTOTHERMAL METHOD

Symptothermal Method is a combination of the BBT and Ovulation Methods.

Information is available from:

Serena
55 Parkdale Avenue
Ottawa, Ontario
K1Y 1E5

(613) 728-6536

## The Parents' Team:

This book started with a chapter on the team of helpers that are available to help the mother through pregnancy. Parents, who get home and feel they need advice or someone to listen to their concerns, should remember that the team is still available to help them with the problems that arise with care of the baby and adjusting to parenthood.

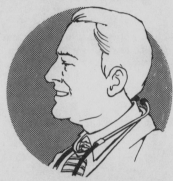

The *physician* continues to provide medical supervision. Any signs or symptoms of illness should be discussed with him. He will also want to see the mother for her postpartum check-up.

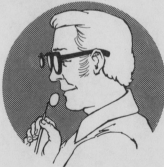

The *dentist* is available to provide care for the new baby as well as for the other members of the family. Although most babies will not cut their first teeth until around the fourth or fifth month, it is important for parents to consider the following guidelines during baby's first weeks and months at home.

a) The dentist should be consulted about fluoride supplements (drops or tablets) and the dosages to be used on a daily basis.
Since fluoride supplements must be continued until at least 14 years of age, it is recommended that a supplement be taken independently of vitamins so that a daily routine can be established. When the child can chew, the "chewable" type of fluoride tablet is recommended.

b) The "Baby Bottle Syndrome" must be prevented. This is decay of early teeth due to sucking on bottles containing sugar-containing liquids or acidic fruit juices, e.g., powdered fruit mixes, fruit juice and milk. The uncontrolled tooth decay can destroy the child's primary teeth by as early as 16 months of age.

c) If a soother is necessary it should never be dipped in a sweet substance such as honey before being put in the baby's mouth.

d) Local irritation of the gums may occur with teething, and the new baby will find it soothing to have the gums cleaned with a 2" x 2" piece of gauze or a wash cloth.

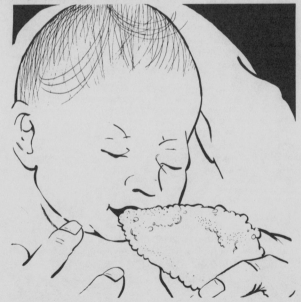

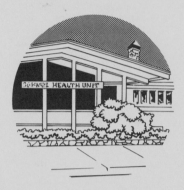

The *health unit's* preventive services become increasingly important to the new parents and baby. The health unit provides a wide range of services including home care, nutrition, dental, speech and hearing and public health inspection.

The *public health nurse* is probably the best known member of the health unit staff to new parents as she is available to discuss concerns that parents may have and also can provide information about other sources of help, some of which are listed inside the front cover of this book. Some concerns parents often bring up during a public health nurse's home visit, in a postnatal or parenting group or at child health conference are:

- breast-feeding
- postnatal exercises
- "blues"
- weight control
- birth control
- family adjustments
- baby's weight
- colic
- formulas
- baby care
- immunization
- postnatal groups
- feelings towards parenthood
- introduction of solids
- baby and child safety

Parents are also invited to phone, drop in or write to their health unit for pamphlets which are available on many baby and toddler topics.

Another member of the health unit team is the public health inspector who may be called upon to test the water of households not on municipal water supply or if water quality is questionable.

The parents and health workers who shared their ideas for this book hope the information has been helpful and ask parents to return the following questionnaire so that their suggestions can be used in the preparation of the next edition of this book.

## NOTES

# NOTES

# SUGGESTED READING FOR PARENTS

## BREAST-FEEDING

Eiger, M.S. and S.W. Olds. *The Complete Book of Breastfeeding.* New York: The Workman Press, 1973.

Ewy, Rodger and Donna. *Preparation for Breastfeeding.* New York: Dolphin Books, 1975.

La Leche League International. *The Womanly Art of Breastfeeding.* Great Britain: Souvenir Press Ltd., 1970.

Pryor, Karen. *Nursing Your Baby.* New York: Harper and Row, 1963.

## CHILDBIRTH

Bean, Constance. *Methods of Childbirth.* Garden City, New York: Doubleday and Company, 1974.

Bing, Elisabeth. *Six Practical Lessons for an Easier Childbirth.* New York: Bantam Books, 1969.

Birkbeck, Adele and Margaret Keen. *Controlled Childbirth.* Vancouver B.C.: J.J. Douglas, 1975.

Bradley, Robert A. *Husband Coached Childbirth.* New York: Harper and Row, 1975.

Dick-Read, Grantley. *Childbirth Without Fear.* New York: Harper and Row Books, 1970.

Ewy, Rodger and Donna. *Preparation for Childbirth.* New York: New American Library, 1970.

Karmel, Marjorie. *Thankyou, Dr. Lamaze.* New York: Dolphin Books, 1965.

Kitzinger, Sheila. *Giving Birth.* New York: Schocken Books, 1977.

Tanzer, Deborah. *Why Natural Childbirth.* New York: Schocken Books, 1976.

## EARLY FAMILY RELATIONSHIPS, PARENTING AND INFANT CARE

Boston Children's Medical Center. *What to Do When There's Nothing to Do.* New York: Dell Publishing Company Inc., 1968.

Brazelton, T. Berry. *Toddlers and Parents.* New York: A Delta Special, 1974.

Brazelton, T. Berry. *Infants and Mothers.* New York: A Delta Book, 1969.

Caplan, Frank. *The First Twelve Months of Life.* New York: Grosset & Dunlap, 1973.

Dodson, Fitzhugh. *How to Father.* New York: New American Library, 1975.

Dreuikers, Rudolph and Vicki Soltz. *Children The Challenge.* New York: Hawthorn Books, 1964.

Ginott, Haim G. *Between Parent and Child; New Solutions to Old Problems.* New York: MacMillan, 1965.

Gordon, Ira. *Baby Learning Through Baby Play.* New York: St. Martin's Press, 1976.

Gordon, Thomas. *Parent Effectiveness Training.* New York: Peter H. Wyden, 1973.

Salk, Lee. *Preparing for Parenthood.* New York: Bantam Books, 1974.

Stein, S.B. *New Parents' Guide to Early Learning.* Scarborough: A Plume Book, 1976.

White, Burton. *First Three Years of Life.* New York: Avon Books, 1975.

## FETAL DEVELOPMENT

Nilsson, Lennart. *A Child is Born.* New York: Delacorte Press, 1966.

Power, Jules. *How Life Begins.* New York: Simon and Schuster, 1965.

## PRENATAL AND INFANT NUTRITION

Kenda, M.E. and P.S. Williams. *The Natural Baby Food Cookbook.* New York: Avon, 1973.

Lambert-Lagace, L. *Feeding Your Child.* Cambridge, Ontario: Collier-Macmillan Canada Ltd., 1976.

Payne, A. *The Baby Food Book.* Toronto: Little, Brown, and Co., Toronto, 1977.

Williams, P.S. *Nourishing Your Unborn Child.* New York: Avon, 1975.

## PREPARING THE CHILDREN

Andry, Andrew C. and Steven Schepp. *How Babies Are Made.* New York: Time-Life Books, 1968.

Sheffield, Margaret. *Where do Babies Come From?* New York: Alfred A. Knopf, 1975.

Showers, Paul and Kay Sperry Showers. *Before You Were a Baby.* Toronto: Fitzhenry and Whiteside Limited, 1968.

## PSYCHOLOGICAL ASPECTS OF CHILDBEARING

Barber, Virginia and M.M. Skaggs. *The Mother Person.* New York: Bobbs-Merrill, 1975.

Colman, Libby and Arthur. *Pregnancy: The Psychological Experience.* New York: Seabury Press, 1971.

Elkins, V.H. *The Rights of the Pregnant Parent.* Ottawa: Waxwing Productions, 1976.

## SEXUAL RELATIONS AND BIRTH CONTROL

Bing, Elisabeth and Libby Colman. *Making Love During Pregnancy.* New York: Bantam Books, 1977.

Kippley, Sheila. *Breastfeeding and Natural Child Spacing.* New York: Penguin Books, 1974.

Rozdilsky, Mary Lou. *What Now? A Handbook for New Parents.* New York: Scribner, 1975.

*IT IS SUGGESTED THAT PARENTS REVIEW THE SELECTION OF PAMPHLETS AT THEIR NEAREST HEALTH UNIT.*

# NOTES

# REFERENCES

## BOOKS

Arms, Suzanne. *A Season to be Born.* New York: Harper and Row, 1973.

Barber, Virginia and Merrill Skaggs. *The Mother Person.* New York: Bobbs-Merrill, 1975.

Beals, Peg, Ed. *Parents' Guide to the Childbearing Year.* Rochester, New York: The International Childbirth Education Association, 1975.

Bean, Constance. *Methods of Childbirth.* New York: Doubleday and Co., 1974.

Benson, Ralph C. *Handbook of Obstetrics and Gynecology.* Los Altos: Lange Medical Publications, 1977.

Bing, Elisabeth. *Adventure of Birth.* New York: Ace Books, 1970.

Bing, Elisabeth. *Moving Through Pregnancy.* Indianapolis: Bobbs-Merrill, 1975.

Bing, Elisabeth. *Six Practical Lessons for an Easier Childbirth.* New York: Bantam Books, 1969.

Bing, E. and L. Colman. *Making Love During Pregnancy.* New York: Bantam Books, 1977.

Birkbeck, Adele and Margaret Keen. *Controlled Childbirth.* Vancouver, B.C.: J.J. Douglas, 1975.

Boston Women's Health Book Collective. *Our Bodies, Ourselves.* New York: Simon and Schuster, 1973.

Boston Children's Medical Center and Richard Feinbloom. *Child Health Encyclopedia.* New York: Dell Publishing Company, 1975.

Bourne, Gordon. *Pregnancy.* London: Pan Books, 1975.

Bowlby, John. *Child Care and the Growth of Love.* London: Penguin Books, 1963.

Bradley, Robert A. *Husband Coached Childbirth.* New York: Harper and Row, 1974.

Brazleton, T. Berry. *Infants and Mothers.* New York: Delacorte Press, 1969.

Brazleton, T. Berry. *Parents and Toddlers.* New York: A Delta Special, 1974.

Canada Department of Health and Welfare. *Oral Contraceptives Report, 1978.* Ottawa, 1978.

Caplan, Frank. *First Twelve Months of Life.* New York: Grosset and Dunlap, 1973.

Castle, Sue. *The Complete Guide to Preparing Baby Foods at Home.* New York: Doubleday and Company, 1973.

Chabon, Irwin. *Awake and Aware.* New York: Dell Publishing Company, 1969.

Clark, Ann L. and Dyanne D. Affonso. *Childbearing: A Nursing Perspective.* Philadelphia: F.A. Davis Co., 1976.

Clausen, Joy Princeton et al. *Maternity Nursing Today.* New York: McGraw-Hill Book Company, 1973.

Colman, Libby and Arthur. *Pregnancy: The Psychological Experience.* New York: Seabury Press, 1971.

Coft, Doreen J. *Be Honest With Yourself.* California: Wadsworth Publishing Company, 1976.

Cruise, Heloise. *Household Hints.* Englewood Cliffs, N.J.: Prentice Hall, Inc., 1962.

Deutsch, Ronald. *Key to Feminine Response in Marriage.* New York: Ballantine, 1968.

Dick-Read, Grantley. *Childbirth Without Fear.* New York: Harper and Row Books, 1970.

Dickason, Elizabeth J. and Martha Olsen Schult, Eds. *Maternal and Infant Care.* New York: McGraw-Hill Inc., 1975.

Dickason, Elizabeth J. et al. Eds. *Maternal and Infant Drugs and Nursing Intervention.* Toronto: McGraw-Hill Book Company, 1978.

Dilfer, Carol S. *Your Baby, Your Body.* New York: Crown Publishers, Inc., 1977.

Dodson, Fitzhugh. *How to Father.* New York: New American Library, 1975.

Dodson, Fitzhugh. *How to Parent.* New York: New American Library, 1973.

Donovan, Bonnie. *The Cesarean Birth Experience.* Boston: Beacon Press, 1977.

Dreikurs, Rudolph. *Children the Challenge.* New York: Hawthorn Books, 1964.

Eastman, Nicholson J. *Expectant Motherhood.* Boston: Little, Brown and Company, 1963.

Eiger, Marvin and Sally Olds. *The Complete Book of Breastfeeding.* New York: Bantam Books, 1973.

Elkins, V.H. *The Rights of the Pregnant Parent.* Ottawa: Waxwing Productions, 1977.

Ewy, Donna and Rodger. *Preparation for Breastfeeding.* New York: Dolphin Books, 1975.

Ewy, Rodger and Donna. *Preparation for Childbirth.* New York: New American Library, 1970.

Flanagan, Geraldine Lux. *The First Nine Months of Life.* New York: Pocket Books, 1962.

Fomon S.J. *Infant Nutrition.* Toronto: W.B. Saunders Company, 1974.

Fromme, Allan. *A.B.C. of Child Care.* New York: Simon and Schuster, 1974.

Genne, William. *Husbands and Pregnancy.* New York: Association Press, 1956.

Gerald, Alice. *Please Breast Feed Your Baby.* New York: New American Library, 1970.

Gesell, Arnold et al. *Infant and Child.* New York: Harper and Row, Publishers, 1974.

Ginott, Haim G. *Between Parent and Child.* New York: MacMillan, 1968.

Goerzen, Janice L. and Peggy L. Chinn. *Review of Maternal and Child Nursing.* St. Louis: C.V. Mosby, 1975.

Good, Ruth. *A Book for Grandmothers.* New York: MacMillan Publishing Company, 1976.

Goodrich, Frederick. *Preparing for Childbirth.* Englewood Cliffs, N.J.: Prentice-Hall, 1966.

Greenblant, M. and M.A. Schucket, Eds. *Alcohol Problems in Women and Children.* New York: Greene and Straton Company, 1976.

Gunther, Mavis. *Infant Feeding.* London: Methuen, 1970.

Guttmacher, Alan. *Pregnancy, Birth and Family Planning.* New York: Viking Press, 1973.

Hassid, Patricia. *Textbook for Childbirth Educators.* Hagerstown, Maryland: Harper and Row, Publishers, 1978.

Hatcher, Robert A. et al. *Contraceptive Technology 1976-1977.* New York: Irvington Publishers, Inc., 1976.

Hazell, Lester. *Commonsense Childbirth.* New York: Berkeley Publishing Corporation, 1976.

Health and Welfare Canada. *Recommended Standards for Maternity and Newborn Care.* Ottawa, 1979.

Hoekelman, Robert A. et al. *Principles of Pediatrics: Health Care of the Young.* New York: McGraw-Hill Inc., 1978.

Homan, William. *Child Sense.* New York: Basic Books, 1977.

Illingworth, R.S. *The Normal Child.* New York: Churchill Livingstone, 1975.

Jacobson, Edmond. *How to Relax and Have Your Baby.* New York: McGraw-Hill, 1959.

Jensen, Margaret Duncan et al. *Maternity Care, The Nurse and the Family.* Saint Louis: The C.V. Mosby Company, 1977.

Karmel, Marjorie. *Thank you, Dr. Lamaze.* Garden City, New York: Dolphin Books, 1959.

Kenda, Margaret E. and Phyllis B. Williams. *The Natural Baby Foods Cookbook.* New York: Avon, 1973.

Kippley, Sheila. *Breastfeeding and Natural Child Spacing.* New York: Penguin Books, 1975.

Kitzinger, Sheila. *Giving Birth.* New York: Schocken Books, 1977.

Kitzinger, Sheila. *The Experience of Childbirth*. Middlesex, England: Penguin Books, 1967.

Klaus, M.H. and J.H. Kennell. *Maternal-Infant Bonding*. St. Louis: The C.V. Mosby Company, 1976.

LaLeche League International. *The Womanly Art of Breastfeeding*. Great Britain: Souvenir Press Ltd., 1970.

Lamaze, Fernand. *Painless Childbirth*. Chicago: Contemporary Books, 1970.

Lambert-Lagace, L. *Feeding Your Child*. Cambridge, Ontario: Collier-Macmillan Canada Ltd., 1976.

Lane, Carolyn and Pamela Zapata. *The Pregnant Cook's Book, or I'm Not Fat I'm Pregnant*. New York: Viking Press, 1970.

Leboyer, Frederick. *Birth Without Violence*. New York: Alfred A. Knopf, 1975.

*Lippincott Manual of Nursing Practice*. Philadelphia: Lippincott, 1978.

Marlow, Dorothy R. *Textbook of Pediatric Nursing*. Philadelphia: W.B. Saunders, 1977.

Masters, William H. and V.E. Johnson. *Human Sexual Response*. Boston: Little, Brown and Company, 1966.

Masters, William H. and V.E. Johnson. *Pleasure Bond*. New York: Bantam Books, 1974.

Maternity Center Association. *A Baby is Born*. New York: Grosset and Dunlap Publishers, 1964.

Miller, John S. *Childbirth: A Manual for Pregnancy and Delivery*. New York: Atheneum, 1974.

Montague, Ashley. *Life Before Birth*. Toronto: Signet Books, 1964.

Montague, Ashley. *Touching*. New York: Columbia University Press, 1971.

National Academy of Science. *Maternal Nutrition and The Course of Pregnancy*. Washington, D.C.: National Academy of Sciences, 1970.

Newton, Niles. *Family Book of Child Care*. New York: Harper and Row, Publishers, 1957.

Nilsson, L. et al. *A Child is Born*. New York: Dell Publishing, 1966.

Noble, Elizabeth. *Essential Exercises for the Childbearing Year*. Boston: Houghton-Mifflin Company, 1976.

Novak, Edmund et al. *Textbook of Gynecology*. Baltimore: Williams and Williams, 1975.

Payne, A. *The Baby Food Book*. Toronto: Little, Brown and Co., 1977.

Phillips, C.R. and J.T. Anzalone. *Fathering*. Saint Louis: C.V. Mosby Company, 1978.

Pillitteri, Adele. *Nursing Care of the Growing Family*. Boston: Little, Brown and Co., 1976.

Prichardt, J.A. and P.C. Macdonald. *Obstetrics*. New York: Appleton-Century-Crofts Company, 1971.

Pryor, Karen. *Nursing Your Baby*. New York: Harper and Row Publishers, 1963.

Reeder, S. et al. *Maternity Nursing*. Philadelphia: J.B. Lippincott Company, 1976.

Rozdililsky, Mary Lou and Barbara Banat. *What Now?* New York: Scribner, 1975.

Rugh, R. and L. Shettles. *From Conception to Birth*. New York: Harper and Row Publishers, 1971.

Salk, Lee. *Preparation for Parenthood*. New York: Bantam Books, 1974.

Salk, Lee. *What Every Child Would Like His Parents to Know*. New York: McKay, 1972.

Salk, Lee and Rita Kramer. *How to Raise a Human Being*. New York: Random Books, 1968.

Sagebeer, Josephine Evans. *Maternal Health Nursing Review*. New York: Arco Publishing Company, Inc., 1975.

Sasmor, Jeanette. *What Every Husband Should Know About Having a Baby*. Chicago: Nelson-Hall, 1972.

Satir, Virginia. *People Making.* Palo Alto, California: Science and Behavior Books, Inc., 1972.

Schaefer, George. *The Expectant Father.* New York: Barnes and Noble, 1972.

Scipien, Gladys M. et al. *Comprehensive Pediatric Nursing.* New York: McGraw-Hill, Inc., 1975.

Schiller, Jack. *Childhood Illness.* New York: Stein and Day, 1974.

Spock, Benjamin. *Baby and Child Care.* Montreal: Pocket Books of Canada, Ltd., 1958.

Stanway, Penny and Andrew. *Breast is Best.* London: Pan Books, 1978.

Stein, Sara Bennett. *New Parents' Guide to Early Learning.* New York: A Plume Book, New American Library, 1976.

Tanzer, Deborah. *Why Natural Childbirth?* New York: Schocken Books, 1976.

Tucker, Tarvez with Elisabeth Bing. *Prepared Childbirth.* Villanova, Pa: Tobey Publishing, 1975.

Vellay, Pierre. *Childbirth Without Pain.* New York: Dutton, 1959.

Wessel, Helen. *Natural Childbirth and the Family.* New York: Harper and Row, Publishers, 1974.

White, Burton. *First Three Years of Life.* New York: Arm Books, 1975.

Williams, Phyllis. *Nourishing Your Unborn Child.* Los Angeles: Nash, 1974.

Wright, Erna. *The New Childbirth.* New York: Pocket Books, 1971.

## ARTICLES AND PAMPHLETS

Anderson, Joan Wester. "What to Do About Newborn Crying", *Life and Health,* 91(6):26-27, June 1976.

Bartle, Bill and Tom Paton. "Effect of Drugs During Pregnancy", *On Continuing Practice,* 5:9-15, May 1978.

*Baths and Babies.* Johnson and Johnson, Ltd., 2155 Boulevard Pie IX, Montreal, Quebec, H1V 2E4, Pamphlet.

Bishop, Cheryl. "Non Prescription Drugs: A Guide to the Pregnant Patient: Part 4", *Canadian Pharmaceutical Journal,* 3(11):385-388, November 1978.

Bishop, Cheryl. "Non Prescription Drugs: A Guide to the Pregnant Patient: Part 5", *Canadian Pharmaceutical Journal,* 3(12):419-420, December 1978.

Cane, Aleta Feinsod. *Frankly Speaking a Pamphlet for Cesarean Couples.* C/SEC Inc., Pamphlet, 1976.

"Cold Injury in the Newborn", National Association for Maternal and Child Welfare, No. 1 South Audley Street, London, W1Y 6J3, Pamphlet, April 1978.

Deibel, Patricia. "Natural Family Planning: Different Methods", *American Journal of Maternal Child Nursing,* 3(3):171-177, May-June 1978.

Dunn, Henry G. "Maternal Cigarette Smoking During Pregnancy and the Child's Subsequent Development: Neurological and Intellectual Maturation to the Age of 6½ Years", *Canadian Journal of Public Health,* 68:43-49, Jan./Feb. 1977.

Holmes, Thomas H. and Richard H. Rahe. "The Social Readjustment Rating Scale", *Journal of Psychosomatic Research,* 11:213-218, April 1967.

*Mother and Baby.* Health and Welfare, Canada, Ottawa, Booklet.

"Neonatal Cold Injury", National Association for Maternal and Child Welfare, No. 1 South Audley Street, London, V1Y 6J3, Pamphlet, April 1978.

"Questions and Answers: Effects on Infant Breastfed by Marijuana - Smoking Mother", *Journal of American Medical Association,* 213:135, July 6, 1970.

"Review of Circumcision", *Briefs,* 39(4):55-58, April 1975.

"Smoking and Pregnancy", Reprinted from: United States Department of Health, Education and Welfare, *The Health Consequences of Smoking; A Report to the Surgeon-General, 1971,* pp. 385-418.

Stortz, Laurie J. "Unprescribed Drug Products and Pregnancy", *Journal of Obstetric and Gynecologic Nursing,* 4:9-13, July-August 1977.

Stott, D.H. "Children in the Womb: The Effects of Stress", *New Society,* 5:329-31, May 1977.

Taggart, Marie-Elizabeth. "A Practical Guide to Successful Breastfeeding", *Canadian Nurse,* 72:25-35, March 1976.

*The First Years of Life,* Books 1 to 8, Milton Keynes, England: Open University Press, 1977.

*Voluntary Sterilization,* Health and Welfare, Canada, Ottawa, Booklet, 1975.

Young, Diony. *Bonding,* International Childbirth Education Association, Inc., New York, Pamphlet, 1978.

## UNPUBLISHED MATERIALS

McConnell, Ian. "Zen and the Art of Diaperhood", Unpublished Article, 1978.

Expectant Parent Class Manuals from the following health units:

Boundary Health Unit, Surrey, B.C.
Cariboo Health Unit, Williams Lake, B.C.
Selkirk Health Unit, Nelson, B.C.
Simon Fraser Health Unit, Coquitlam, B.C.
South Okanagan Health Unit, Kelowna, B.C.
West Kootenay Health Unit, Trail, B.C.

# GLOSSARY

*abortion*  Termination of a pregnancy before the fetus is viable, usually before 20 weeks gestation (the weight of the fetus or embryo is less than 500 grams). An accidental or spontaneous abortion is often called a miscarriage.

*afterpains*  Uterine cramps due to contraction of the uterus occurring during the first few days after childbirth. The pains are more noticeable in multiparae and may occur during breast-feeding.

*amniocentesis*  A procedure for the removal of some of the amniotic fluid from the amniotic sac by inserting a needle through the abdominal and uterine walls of the mother for the purpose of removing fluid for laboratory studies.

*amniotic fluid*  Fluid surrounding the fetus in the uterus.

*amniotomy*  Approaching the amniotic sac through the vagina and rupturing the sac by artificial means.

*analgesic*  A drug or agent which relieves pain.

*anemia*  Deficiency of hemoglobin or of red blood cells.

*anesthesia*  Partial or complete absence of sensation with or without loss of consciousness.

*antenatal*  Occurring or formed before birth.

*Apgar score*  A system for rating the depression of a newborn infant, at 60 seconds and usually also at 5 and sometimes 10 minutes after birth. The heart rate, respirations, muscle tone, color, and response to stimuli are each scored 0, 1 or 2. The maximum score for a baby is 10, indicating complete absence of depression.

*Braxton Hicks contractions*  Painless, intermittent contractions of the uterus which occur throughout pregnancy; often mistaken for labor contractions.

*breech*  Presentation of the fetus when the buttocks and/or feet are closest to the cervix and will be born before the head.

*circumcision*  Surgical removal of the foreskin (prepuce).

*colostrum*  Yellowish-white fluid secreted by the breasts before, and for the first 2 - 3 days after delivery.

*conception*  Union of the sperm and ovum which results in fertilization.

*congenital*  Present or existing before birth.

*crowning*  Stage of delivery when the largest diameter of the baby's head can be seen through the external opening of the vagina.

*diaphragm*  Muscular wall which is important for breathing. It separates the upper chest cavity (containing the heart and lungs) from the abdominal cavity.

*edema*  A condition in which the body tissues contain an excessive amount of tissue fluid.

*embryo*  Stage in prenatal development after fertilization but prior to development of fetus; that is, between the second and eighth weeks (inclusive) of gestation.

*endometrium*  Mucous membrane which lines the uterus.

*engagement*  Descent of the uterus into the pelvic cavity as the presenting part of the fetus settles into the pelvis.

*episiotomy*  Incision (cut) often made in the perineum at the end of the second stage of labor to enlarge the opening of the vagina.

*exchange transfusion*  Replacement of 70% to 80% of the baby's circulating blood and injecting the donor's blood in equal amounts.

*fetus*   Name given the developing baby from the beginning of the ninth week of gestation until birth.

*fontanels*   ("soft spots")   Areas consisting of strong connective tissue at the junctions of the cranial (skull) bones of the baby.

*forceps*   A tong-like instrument used to facilitate the delivery of the baby's head through the lower pelvis.

*foreskin*   (prepuce)   Loose fold of skin covering the end of the penis.

*fundus*   The upper muscular part of the uterus.

*gestation*   Period of development from fertilization of the ovum to birth.

*gestational age*   The number of completed weeks/days of fetal development counting from the first day of the last normal menstrual cycle.

*gravida*   A pregnant woman. Primagravida refers to a woman who is pregnant for the first time; multigravida, to a woman who has been pregnant more than once.

*hemoglobin*   Hemo (iron-containing pigment)   globulin (a simple protein). Its function is to carry oxygen to the tissues.

*induction*   The use of drugs or procedures to inititate the onset of labor.

*involution*   The return of the uterus after delivery to its non-pregnant weight and shape.

*jaundice*   A condition characterized by yellowish discoloration of the skin and other body tissues caused by deposit of bile pigments.

*lactation*   Secretion of milk from the mammary glands, or the period during which milk is secreted.

*lightening*   Sensation of decreased abdominal distention as a result of engagement.

*lochia*   Uterine discharge of blood, mucus and tissue through the vagina during the puerperium.

*low birth weight*   Refers to fetuses or infants weighing less than 2,500 grams at birth, whether or not born preterm.

*mammary glands*   The glands of the female breast that secrete milk.

*meconium*   The material which forms as the intestinal content of the fetus and which apears as the newborn's first stools. It is greenish-brown or black and sticky.

*molding*   Temporary shaping of the fetal head to fit through the mother's birth canal during labor.

*neonate*   Newborn from birth to 28 days of life.

*os*   Opening.

*palpation*   Examination by touching the external surface of the body with the fingers or palm of the hand such as feeling the abdominal wall to detect the position of the fetus.

*parity*   Refers to having given birth to a live or stillborn infant; primipara means a woman giving birth for the first time; multipara refers to a woman who has given birth before.

*perineum*   Area between the vagina and the rectum in the female and between the scrotum and rectum in the male.

*postmature·baby*   Infant born at the beginning of the 42nd week of gestation or later.

*premature*   A confusing term sometimes applied to low birth-weight infants (under 2,500 grams) and sometimes applied to infants born before term, i.e. before completion of 37 weeks of gestation.

*presentation*   (presenting part)   The part of the fetus which lies closest to the opening of the cervix.

*preterm infant*    An infant born before completion of 37 weeks after the first day of the last menstrual period.

*prolapsed cord*    Protrusion of the umbilical cord ahead of the presenting part of the fetus.

*puerperium*    Period of time after delivery of the baby and placenta until involution of uterus occurs (approximately 6 weeks).

*resuscitation*    Restoration of breathing, life or consciousness in one whose respirations had ceased.  In the case of resuscitation of the newborn baby, resuscitation involves blowing oxygen into the lungs for each breath when the baby's own breathing efforts are absent or inadequate, and occasionally assisting the heart contractions as well.

*surfactant* (pulmonary)    A substance produced by the lungs and necessary to prevent collapse of the air sacs (alveoli) by surface tension.

*toxemia* (now called pre-eclampsia − eclampsia)    Condition sometimes occurring in the mother during pregnancy or the puerperium. Most common signs are edema, increased blood pressure and sudden weight gain.

*transition breathing*    A rhythmic pattern of shallow breathing and short puff blows.

*trimester*    Period of three months; pregnancy is divided into 1st, 2nd and 3rd trimesters as an approximation of gestational age which is expressed in weeks or days.

*vernix*    A grayish-white cheeselike substance which usually covers and protects skin of the fetus and the newborn infant.

*vertex*    Refers to the crown or top of the head.  Vertex presentation describes the position of the fetus when the skull is nearest the cervix.  When the head is born first, the birth is called a vertex delivery.

*viable*    Capable of living, as a newborn or fetus which has reached a stage that will permit it to live outside the uterus.

*zygote*    The fertilized ovum.

116

# INDEX

## QUESTIONNAIRE

Please circle the chapters of this book that you read: all, 1, 2, 3, 4, 5, 6, 7, 8, 9.

What parts were unclear?

What additional topics should have been included?

What topics could have been omitted?

Other comments:

It is not necessary to sign this questionnaire but if signed, your suggestions will be acknowledged.

Name . . . . . . . . . . . . . . . . . . . . . . . . . . . . . . . . . . . . . . . . . . . . . . . . . . . . . .

Address . . . . . . . . . . . . . . . . . . . . . . . . . . . . . . . . . . . . . . . . . . . . . . . . . . .

Please mail directly or take to your nearest health unit for forwarding to:

Public Health Nursing Division
B.C. Ministry of Health
1515 Blanshard Street
Victoria, B.C.
V8W 3C8